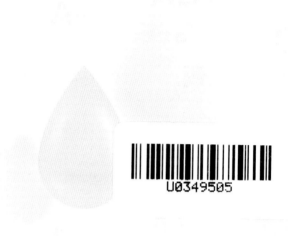

U0349505

2018 年
国家血液安全报告

China's Report on Blood Safety 2018

国家卫生健康委员会　编

National Health Commission of the People's Republic of China

人民卫生出版社

图书在版编目（CIP）数据

2018 年国家血液安全报告 / 国家卫生健康委员会编
. —北京：人民卫生出版社，2020
ISBN 978-7-117-29989-3

Ⅰ.①2… Ⅱ.①国… Ⅲ.①输血 – 卫生管理 – 研究
报告 – 中国 –2018 Ⅳ.①R457.1

中国版本图书馆 CIP 数据核字（2020）第 074425 号

人卫智网	www.ipmph.com	医学教育、学术、考试、健康，购书智慧智能综合服务平台
人卫官网	www.pmph.com	人卫官方资讯发布平台

本书中所有地图审图号：GS（2020）954 号

2018 年国家血液安全报告

编　　写：国家卫生健康委员会
出版发行：人民卫生出版社（中继线 010-59780011）
地　　址：北京市朝阳区潘家园南里 19 号
邮　　编：100021
E - mail：pmph @ pmph.com
购书热线：010-59787592　010-59787584　010-65264830
印　　刷：北京顶佳世纪印刷有限公司
经　　销：新华书店
开　　本：710×1000　1/16　　印张：19
字　　数：351 千字
版　　次：2020 年 6 月第 1 版　2020 年 6 月第 1 版第 1 次印刷
标准书号：ISBN 978-7-117-29989-3
定　　价：98.00 元
打击盗版举报电话：010-59787491　E-mail：WQ @ pmph.com
质量问题联系电话：010-59787234　E-mail：zhiliang @ pmph.com

编写工作组名单

主编 张宗久

主审 郭燕红　焦雅辉　周长强　邢若齐

编委 高新强　张　睿　陈　斌　冷婷婷　胡　翔　王　毅
姚德明　李大川　马旭东　刘　勇　陈　虎　黄　欣

编写组专家（按姓氏笔画排序）

王　岚　武汉血液中心

王　明　福建省血液中心

王　娅　中国医学科学院输血研究所

王兆福　河南省红十字血液中心

王相荣　吉林省血液中心

王常虹　甘肃省红十字血液中心

王露楠　国家卫生健康委临床检验中心

邓晓林　贵州省血液中心

付涌水　广州血液中心

白　林　山西省血液中心

冯　凌　云南昆明血液中心

朱为刚　深圳市血液中心

刘　江　北京市红十字血液中心

刘　忠　中国医学科学院输血研究所

刘存旭　广西壮族自治区血液中心

刘爱民　中国医学科学院输血研究所

刘嘉馨　中国医学科学院输血研究所
孙　光　黑龙江省血液中心
孙　俊　江苏省血液中心
纪宏文　中国医学科学院阜外医院
严力行　浙江省血液中心
李恒新　陕西省血液中心
汪传喜　广州血液中心
汪德清　中国人民解放军总医院
宋秀宇　厦门市中心血站
张荣江　天津市血液中心
张洪斌　乌鲁木齐血液中心
张新童　山东省血液中心
陆韬宏　上海市血液中心
范文安　安徽省血液管理中心
范为民　江西省血液中心
赵　楠　内蒙古自治区血液中心
赵生银　宁夏血液中心
胡　伟　浙江省血液中心
胡晓玉　安徽省血液中心
逄淑涛　青岛市中心血站
夏　荣　复旦大学附属华山医院
徐　红　宁波市中心血站
郭永建　福建省血液中心
宴永和　湖南省血液中心
戚　海　河北省血液中心
符策瑛　海南省血液中心
梁晓华　大连市血液中心
董晓蓉　西藏自治区血液中心
傅雪梅　成都市血液中心
戴苏娜　中国输血协会

前　言

　　2018年是《中华人民共和国献血法》(以下简称《献血法》)颁布实施20周年。20年来,我国无偿献血法制化建设不断完善,采供血服务体系不断健全,血液供应基本保证,血液安全有力保障。2018年,我国血液安全工作以"提升依法治理水平、提升血液供应水平、提升血液安全水平、提升合理用血水平"为主线,着力构建了"来源可靠、公平可及、全程质控、使用合理"的血液安全保障体系。

一、血液安全法治化管理水平不断提升

　　截至2018年,我国各省(自治区、直辖市)都制定并实施了《献血法》实施条例或办法,13个省会城市和14个独立立法权城市颁布了市级的献血条例或办法。初步形成了国家、省、市三级无偿献血法制化体系建设,确保血液安全管理工作有法可依、有章可循。在血液安全技术标准体系建设中,2018年基本完成了标准体系的框架设计,同时发布了4项卫生行业标准,血液技术标准体系不断健全和完善。

二、无偿献血激励机制不断创新

　　全国各地不断探索无偿献血激励机制,积极拓展无偿献血宣传与招募模式。国家卫生健康委员会、中国红十字会总会、中央军委后勤保障部卫生局首次推出4名国家无偿献血宣传员,以弘扬无偿献血救死扶伤的人道主义精神。同时,在《献血法》实施20周年之际,对全国表现突出的304个采血班组予以通报表扬。各省(自治区、直辖市)紧密结合当地特色,部门之间协调联动,创新无偿献血宣传教育模式和献血者权益保障措施,积极推进无偿献血者临床用血费用和异地用血费用减免管理办法,营造了良好的无偿献血社会氛围。

三、采供血服务体系不断优化

　　2018年,全国血站使用面积和建筑面积等基础条件不断优化,占地总面

积约 216 万 m^2,较 2017 年增加 2.70%;献血点和送血车等服务设施持续增加,献血点数量达到 1 458 个,较 2017 年增长 5.65%。实验室检测和血液制备等仪器设备不断升级、血站从业人员结构不断优化,高学历从业人员和卫生技术人员占比持续增加。信息化建设日益完善,26 个省份实现了血站与献血点之间的全程联网,逐步建立了从血管到血管的覆盖采供血全过程的血液质量管理信息系统。

四、血液供应保障能力持续提升

2018 年我国无偿献血总人次、献血总量和千人口献血率又创新高,分别达到 1 479 万人次、2 506 万 U 和 11.1‰。全国血液成分分离率达 99.82%;红细胞类成分供应量 2 260.7 万 U,比 2017 年增长 2.8%;单采血小板 177.9 万 U,比 2017 年增长 10.2%;血浆类成分达到 2 132.2 万 U,比 2017 年增长 12.4%。2018 年,西藏自治区血液中心自主开展血液核酸检测,填补了我国西藏地区没有核酸检测实验室的空白,有力地保障了当地血液安全。

(注:本书数据不含我国港澳台地区)

编者
2020 年 1 月

目　录

第一篇　血液安全法制建设 ……………………………………………… 1

　第一章　血液管理法制建设 …………………………………………… 2

　第二章　输血行业标准制定 …………………………………………… 6

第二篇　无偿献血社会氛围 ……………………………………………… 9

　第一章　无偿献血宣传 ………………………………………………… 11

　第二章　无偿献血促进 ………………………………………………… 15

　第三章　无偿献血志愿服务 …………………………………………… 19

第三篇　血站建设与发展 ………………………………………………… 25

　第一章　从业人员 ……………………………………………………… 27

　第二章　基础设施 ……………………………………………………… 31

　第三章　信息化建设 …………………………………………………… 34

第四篇　献血招募与血液采集 …………………………………………… 37

　第一章　献血模式 ……………………………………………………… 38

　第二章　献血人群 ……………………………………………………… 41

　第三章　血液采集 ……………………………………………………… 44

第五篇　血液检测和质量保证 …………………………………………… 49

　第一章　血站血液检测 ………………………………………………… 50

　第二章　室间质量评价 ………………………………………………… 56

　第三章　质量保证 ……………………………………………………… 63

第六篇　血液供应和临床用血 …………………………………………… 65

　第一章　血液成分供应 ………………………………………………… 66

第二章　临床用血 ………………………………………………………… 72

第七篇　单采血浆站 ………………………………………………………… 81

第八篇　输血医学科研与教育 ……………………………………………… 85

第一章　输血医学科研 …………………………………………………… 86
第二章　输血医学教育 …………………………………………………… 91
第三章　学术交流与国际合作 …………………………………………… 93

第九篇　不断发展的西藏采供血事业 ……………………………………… 95

第十篇　总结与展望 ………………………………………………………… 101

第一章　主要成绩 ………………………………………………………… 102
第二章　面临的挑战 ……………………………………………………… 105
第三章　展望 ……………………………………………………………… 106

附录 …………………………………………………………………………… 109

附表 1　2018 年千人口献血率汇总表 …………………………………… 109
附表 2　2018 年血液采集情况汇总表 …………………………………… 110
附表 3　2018 年个人献血比例汇总表 …………………………………… 112
附表 4　2018 年 400ml 献血占比情况汇总表 …………………………… 113
附表 5　2018 年女性献血者比例汇总表 ………………………………… 114
附表 6　2018 年 18~35 岁献血者占比情况汇总表 ……………………… 115
附表 7　2018 年本科以上学历献血者占比情况汇总表 ………………… 116
附表 8　2018 年血站血液检测情况汇总表 ……………………………… 117
附表 9　2018 年献血前检测结果汇总表 ………………………………… 118
附表 10　2018 年血液实验室检测情况汇总表 ………………………… 119
附表 11　2018 年血液成分分离比例情况汇总表 ……………………… 121
附表 12　2018 年浓缩血小板分离率汇总表 …………………………… 122
附表 13　2018 年供血总量汇总表 ……………………………………… 123
附表 14　2018 年万人血小板使用量汇总表 …………………………… 124
附表 15　2018 年有形成分利用率汇总表 ……………………………… 125
附表 16　2018 年血液物理报废汇总表 ………………………………… 126
附表 17　2018 年各主要城市血液采集情况 …………………………… 127

Contents

Section One   Legislative Development for Blood Safety·······135
Chapter One   Legislative Development for Blood Management ···············136
Chapter Two   Formulating Industry Standards for Blood Transfusion ··········143

Section Two   Social Awareness of Voluntary
Non-Remunerated Blood Donation ···················147
Chapter One   Publicity of Voluntary Non-remunerated Blood Donation ·······149
Chapter Two   Promotion of Voluntary Non-remunerated Blood Donation·····155
Chapter Three   Voluntary Non-remunerated Blood Donation ····················161

Section Three   Development and Operation of Blood Centers···· 167
Chapter One   Employees ···169
Chapter Two   Infrastructure ···175
Chapter Three   Informatization Building ·······································180

Section Four   The Recruitment of Blood Donors and Blood
Collection ··183
Chapter One   Blood Donation Types···184
Chapter Two   Donor Backgrounds ··187
Chapter Three   Blood Collection ···190

Section Five   Blood Testing and Quality Assurance ···············195
Chapter One   Blood Testing at Blood Centers ································196
Chapter Two   External Quality Assessment of Laboratories··················203
Chapter Three   Quality Assurance ···211

Section Six   Blood Supply and Blood for Clinical Use···········215
Chapter One   Blood Components Supply······································216
Chapter Two   Blood for Clinical Use··222

Section Seven   Plasmapheresis Centers ···235

Section Eight   Transfusion Medicine: Research and
                 Education ···239
Chapter One   Transfusion Medicine: Research and Education ·····················240
Chapter Two   Transfusion Medicine Education ·································246
Chapter Three   Academic Exchange and International Cooperation ···············248

Section Nine   The Continuous Development of Blood Collection
                 and Supply in Xizang Zizhiqu ································251

Section Ten   Conclusion and Future Prospects·················259
Chapter One   Main Achievements···260
Chapter Two   Challenges ···264
Chapter Three   Future Prospects···266

Appendices··269
Appendix 1   Summary of blood donation pate per 1,000
                 population in 2018 ··269
Appendix 2   Summary of the volume of blood donation in 2018···············270
Appendix 3   Summary of individual blood donation rate in 2018···············272
Appendix 4   Summary of 400ml blood donation rate in 2018 ·················273
Appendix 5   Summary of female blood donor rate in 2018 ···················274
Appendix 6   Summary of blood donation rate aged 18 to 35 in 2018···········275
Appendix 7   Summary of blood donation rate with bachelor degree
                 or above in 2018 ··276
Appendix 8   Summary of blood testing at blood centers in 2018···············277
Appendix 9   Summary of pre-donation blood screening in 2018 ···············279
Appendix 10   Summary of blood laboratory testing at blood
                 centers in 2018 ··281
Appendix 11   Summary of blood component separation rate in 2018···········283
Appendix 12   Summary of concentrated platelet separation rate in 2018·······284
Appendix 13   Summary of total blood supply volume in 2018·················285
Appendix 14   Summary of platelet use volume (10,000 people) in 2018·······286
Appendix 15   Summary of tangible components utilization rate in 2018·······287
Appendix 16   Summary of physical discarded blood in 2018·················288
Appendix 17   Summary of blood collection in major cities in 2018 ···········290

第一篇

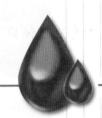

血液安全
法制建设

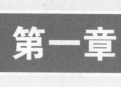

第一章

血液管理法制建设

一、地方立法体系不断完善,血液安全法治建设有力保障

《献血法》的颁布实施,使我国血液管理工作步入法制化轨道。为贯彻实施《献血法》,各省市地方立法相继开展,围绕《献血法》实施的地方立法体系不断完善。逐步形成国家《献血法》、省级"实施《献血法》条例"、地市"落实相应条例办法"的三级法制化体系建设。

自 1998 年《献血法》颁布实施以来,截至 2018 年,全国有 31 个省(自治区、直辖市)颁布了《献血法》实施条例或办法,其中北京、河北、上海、浙江、山东、广东、广西、海南共计 8 省(自治区、直辖市)就地方立法进行了第一次修订,江苏、重庆进行了第二次修订。2018 年海南启动第一次修订工作,广东和重庆于2017 年完成修订工作并于 2018 年施行(表 1-1)。

表 1-1　部分地方立法修法情况一览表

序号	地区	法规名称	颁布时间	修订情况	
				第一次 修订时间	第二次 修订时间
1	北京	北京市公民献血用血管理办法 / 北京市献血管理办法	1999	2009	—
2	河北	河北省实施《中华人民共和国 献血法》办法	2000	2010	—
3	上海	上海市献血条例	1998	2010	—
4	江苏	江苏省献血条例	2000	2010	2017

序号	地区	法规名称	颁布时间	修订情况	
				第一次修订时间	第二次修订时间
5	浙江	浙江省实施《中华人民共和国献血法》办法	2001	2013	—
6	山东	山东省实施《中华人民共和国献血法》办法	2000	2004	—
7	广东	广东省实施《中华人民共和国献血法》办法	1998	2017	—
8	广西	广西壮族自治区献血条例	2001	2010	
9	海南	海南经济特区无偿献血条例	2012	2018(启动)	
10	重庆	重庆市献血条例	1998	2010	2017

在省级立法的推动下,各地方落实《献血法》办法或相应条例等立法工作也相继展开。截至 2018 年,全国省会城市中有乌鲁木齐、西安、杭州、济南等 13 个省会城市颁布了市级落实《献血法》办法,其中西安、沈阳和南宁的立法已进行了第一次修订,昆明的立法已进行了第二次修订(表 1-2)。有力地保证了地方贯彻落实《献血法》,血液安全得到了有力的保障。各级地方立法为血液安

表 1-2　省会城市立法情况(按颁布时间排序)

序号	城市	法规名称	颁布时间	修订时间
1	乌鲁木齐	乌鲁木齐市公民义务献血条例	1993	已废止
2	西安	西安市实施《中华人民共和国献血法》办法	1998	2013
3	杭州	杭州市实施《中华人民共和国献血法》办法	1999	—
4	济南	济南市献血管理若干规定	2001	—
5	沈阳	沈阳市献血管理办法	2001	2016
6	武汉	武汉市献血条例	2002	
7	昆明	昆明市献血用血管理办法 昆明市献血条例	2002	2008 2018
8	广州	广州市献血管理规定	2004	—
9	南宁	南宁市献血条例	2004	2012
10	成都	成都市《中华人民共和国献血法》实施办法	2011	—
11	贵阳	贵阳市公民用血管理办法	2011	—
12	太原	太原市献血条例	2015	
13	南京	南京市献血条例	2017	—

全法治化建设提供了有力保障。

　　全国 22 个有独立立法权的城市中有 14 个颁布该地区的献血条例或办法，其中青岛、厦门、抚顺、苏州、徐州、宁波、唐山已进行了第一次修订，也有部分城市因立法时间较早而废止，如淄博和大连（表 1-3）。

表 1-3　独立立法权城市立法情况（按颁布时间排序）

序号	城市	法规名称	颁布时间	最新修订时间
1	齐齐哈尔	齐齐哈尔市公民献血和血液管理条例	1996	—
2	青岛	青岛市公民义务献血条例	1996	2003
3	淄博	淄博市公民无偿献血管理办法	1997	2010（废止）
4	厦门	厦门经济特区无偿献血条例	1997	2009
5	抚顺	抚顺市实施《中华人民共和国献血法》暂行办法	1998	2002
6	苏州	苏州市献血条例	1999	2015
7	无锡	无锡市献血管理办法	1999	
8	徐州	徐州市无偿献血条例	1999	2015
9	宁波	宁波市献血条例	1999	2012
10	大连	大连市献血条例	2000	2010（废止）
11	唐山	唐山市献血用血条例	2004	2010
12	大同	大同市献血条例	2007	—
13	吉林	吉林市无偿献血条例	2014	
14	深圳	深圳经济特区无偿献血条例	2015	

二、地方立法内容不断创新，血液安全保障能力不断提高

　　2018 年，部分省份针对血液安全保障工作面临的挑战和存在的问题，从顶层设计和工作机制上开展探索和创新，各级地方立法工作呈现出新的亮点。

　　一是进一步明确政府及相关部门职责。进一步增强了依法执业的可行性和有效性。例如《海南经济特区无偿献血条例》（以下简称《海南条例》）中明确了各级人民政府、财政部门、公安机关和城市管理部门、交通运输管理部门、教育部门、人力资源和社会保障等相关部门在无偿献血工作中的职责。《昆明市献血条例》（以下简称《昆明条例》）明确了市、县（区）人民政府对献血工作的领导将纳入年度责任目标考核，同时明确了各相关部门的工作职责。

　　二是进一步强化无偿献血的社会氛围。《海南条例》规定"每年一月为本

经济特区无偿献血宣传月"。《昆明条例》规定"每年 1 月为医务人员无偿献血月,2 月为公务员无偿献血月。其他无偿献血月由市人民政府确定。"

三是进一步保障献血者权益。《海南条例》规定无偿献血者及其亲属享有优先用血权,"在保证临床急救用血的前提下,对在本经济特区参加无偿献血的公民及其配偶、父母、子女,医疗机构应当优先安排临床用血。"对符合条件的献血者和志愿者可享受"三免"待遇,"在本经济特区献血并获得国家无偿献血奉献奖、国家无偿捐献造血干细胞奖和国家无偿献血志愿服务终身荣誉奖的个人可以凭相关证件,在该经济特区内享受以下优待:(一)免交进入国有资金投资建设的旅游景区景点参观游览门票费;(二)免交公立医疗机构门诊挂号费和诊查费;(三)免费乘坐城市轨道交通和公共汽车;(四)省人民政府规定的其他优待措施"。《昆明条例》规定符合条件的献血者和志愿者可享受"三优四免一补"待遇,"(一)同等条件下优先提供就业岗位,优先推荐就业,优先保障子女入托、入学;(二)免费游览政府投资主办的公园、旅游风景区等场所,免交公立医疗机构普通门诊诊查费,享受优先诊疗,享受每年一次由用血医疗机构提供的基本项目免费健康体检,免费乘坐城市轨道交通和公共汽车;(三)对符合条件的灵活就业人员给予相应社保补贴。"

四是突破和创新。海南作为全国唯一的省级经济特区,在立法上有较大的灵活自主性,在条例修订过程中,结合本地区的特点,开展了一些突破和创新。一是将献血年龄放宽至 65 周岁,规定"既往无献血反应,符合健康检查要求的献血者要求再次献血的,年龄可延长至六十五周岁"。二是调整献血间隔期,规定"两次采集间隔期男性不得少于三个月、女性不得少于四个月"。三是将自体输血费用纳入医保,规定"用血者自体输血发生的费用,按照有关规定纳入基本医疗保险支付范围"。条例的修订极大提升了无偿献血者和志愿者的荣誉感和获得感,不仅让广大献血者切实感受到社会的关爱,更发挥了示范带头作用,进一步调动了健康适龄公民自愿参与无偿献血的积极性。

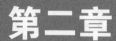

第二章

输血行业标准制定

自 1996 年国家卫生标准委员会血液标准专业委员会成立以来,我国血液标准化工作不断进步。目前已有 2 项国家标准,10 项行业标准(表 1-4)。

表 1-4　血液标准

类型	标准名称
国家标准	《献血者健康检查要求》(GB 18467—2011)
	《全血及成分血质量要求》(GB 18469—2012)
行业标准	《输血医学常用术语》(WS/T 203—2001)
	《献血场所配置要求》(WS/T 401—2012)
	《血液储存要求》(WS 399—2012)
	《血液运输要求》(WS/T 400—2012)
	《全血及成分血质量监测指南》(WS/T 550—2017)
	《献血不良反应分类指南》(WS/T 551—2017)
	《献血相关血管迷走神经反应预防和处置指南》(WS/T 595—2018)
	《内科输血》(WS/T 622—2018)
	《全血和成分血使用》(WS/T 623—2018)
	《输血反应分类》(WS/T 624—2018)

一、血液标准体系框架基本形成

血液标准体系建立是实现采供血和临床输血标准化管理的基础,促进输血行业的发展和技术的进步。根据 2018 年新修订的《中华人民共和国标准化法》,在原有的血液标准体系框架基础上,从血液基础、献血服务、血液制备、血液供应、血液检测、临床输血、质量管理和输血服务信息化共八个方面重新构建了反映标准体系总体组成和层次结构关系的血液标准体系框架,进一步提高血液标准的系统性、协调性和适用性。其中,2018 年发布的 4 项行业标准,《献血相关血管迷走神经反应预防和处置指南》为献血服务方面,《全血和成分血使用》《内科输血》和《输血反应分类》为临床输血方面。同时,血液制备等标准正在持续推进中。血液标准专业委员会对体系框架实行动态管理,根据国际血液行业标准化的最新发展动态,适时进行调整和完善,促进我国血液标准体系结构化、系统化。

二、血液标准制定科学性不断提升

我国血液标准化体系建设不断发展,逐步形成了"政府主导、行业参与、符合国情、对标国际"的标准制定模式和"观点有依据、数据有出处"的标准编制要求。通过参考国外相关标准与针对性、专业性和科学性的调查研究,标准的制定日益规范、科学和合理。2018 年发布的《献血相关血管迷走神经反应预防和处置指南》作为血站业务工作的又一标准,对献血不良反应易发人群的识别、预防和处置措施、人员和设施做出明确要求,为血站工作人员在实际工作中对献血相关不良反应的预防和处置提供了理论基础和技术指导。《全血和成分血使用》是我国第一部血液使用标准,编制专家组开展了三年多的研究,参考了大量国内外相关标准,对全血和成分血的适应证、输注剂量和使用方法、输血反应的分类等做出全新更加科学、合理的要求和规定,标志着我国血液使用迈入标准化的阶段。《内科输血》和《输血反应分类》也是指导临床用血的卫生行业标准。这三个卫生行业标准的发布对进一步促进医疗机构临床输血治疗与评价、临床合理用血有着重要的指导意义,同时为卫生健康行政部门管理督导与评审提供依据。血液相关标准的不断更新和完善,能够更好地规范和指导执业行为,促进行业发展。

2018 年国家血液安全报告

China's Report on Blood Safety 2018

第二篇

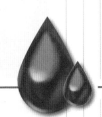

无偿献血
社会氛围

2018 年,国家卫生健康委发布《关于组织开展 2018 年"世界献血者日"宣传活动的通知》(国卫办医函〔2018〕238 号)和《关于开展〈献血法〉实施 20 周年总结宣传活动的通知》(国卫办医函〔2018〕483 号),全国各地积极展开宣传与招募,营造良好的舆论氛围。无偿献血工作得到全社会的广泛理解和热情支持,越来越多富有爱心的公众加入到无偿献血者队伍中来,事业发展呈现出健康、可持续的良好态势。

第一章

无偿献血宣传

一、无偿献血公益宣传日渐活跃

2018 年 6 月 14 日,由国家卫生健康委员会、中国红十字会总会、中央军委后勤保障部卫生局发布的第 15 个"世界献血者日"宣传海报正式公布,海霞、吴京、张翰、菅纫姿作为国家无偿献血宣传员正式亮相。国家卫生健康委员会、中国红十字会总会、中央军委后勤保障部卫生局还联合录制了无偿献血宣传公益广告片,推动无偿献血公益事业健康稳步发展。"献血,赠送生命的礼物""无偿献血,你也可以做他人的英雄""伸出臂膀的那一刻,你就是人群中的聚光点"等一批宣传口号先后推出。受国家卫生健康委的委托,武汉承办了世界献血者日中国主会场活动。

伴随着国家层面无偿献血公益宣传的不断展开,各省积极响应,一方面通过报纸、电台、电视台、海报、车载广告等传统媒体大力宣传无偿献血先进人物和典型事迹,弘扬献血救人的奉献精神和社会正能量。一方面又通过互联网、微信、微博等新媒体扩大受众范围,创新模式,拓宽渠道,以公众喜闻乐见的方式构建出全方位立体传播的体系。通过对全国 27 个省份开展无偿献血促进调研,反馈数据显示所有血站均开设公开日,其中海南省公开日频率更是达到了一月多次,方便公众参观了解献血知识;26 个省份开展了个人先进事迹宣传活动;19 个省份推选了无偿献血大使,其中江西省开展第三届热血英雄传递洪城之爱暨纪念《献血法》实施 20 周年活动,以献血知识答题竞赛的方式评选出 30 位无偿献血传播大使。多省制作无偿献血微电影和宣传片,受到青少年群体的广泛关注。

二、无偿献血宣传活动精彩纷呈

2018 年是《献血法》颁布 20 周年,各省份围绕《献血法》20 周年开展了系列活动,持续推进无偿献血宣传,营造无偿献血良好的社会氛围。各省份在省委、省政府的大力支持下,不断推进"进机关、进企业、进学校、进农村、进社区"的宣传招募形式。其中内蒙古自治区部分盟市将无偿献血宣传活动纵向延伸到牧场、马场,"因地制宜"地开展无偿献血志愿者招募工作。部分地区采取无偿献血知识讲座、现身说教以及无偿献血知识竞赛等创新模式,强化无偿献血宣传教育,弘扬救死扶伤人道主义精神。根据对 26 个省份的无偿献血促进调研结果显示,所有省份均开通了献血专线;20 个省份开展调研了城市人口和在校学生无偿献血知晓率。各省(自治区、直辖市)20 周年宣传活动详见表 2-1。

表 2-1　各省(自治区、直辖市)20 周年宣传活动

地区	活动
黑龙江	开展进校园、进社区、进机关、进企业、进农村宣传 150 余场次活动 在主流载体刊登我省 27 位荣获国家无偿献血志愿者终身荣誉奖事迹报道 全省高校广泛开展以"众志成城二十载、热血汇聚中华情"为主题的无偿献血进校园献血宣传活动
青海	围绕健康青海建设、深化医改等主题,开展多种形式的宣传和报道工作,全年共报送各类信息 106 篇 "无偿献血,你就是英雄"等主题宣传活动
福建	"众志成城二十载,热血汇聚中华情"主题宣传教育活动
湖南	开展演讲比赛、学术研讨班、文艺汇演、气排球赛等活动,发布了汇报片、纪念册、影集等
湖北	承办"闪耀的红"全国血站汇报演讲活动
海南	将修订《海南经济特区无偿献血条例》纳入立法计划 健康热血跑活动
江苏	全省各地采供血机构"五进"宣传次数累计达到 2 500 余场次 "浓浓献血情　心系你我他"为主题的全省无偿献血宣传月活动 "听我说故事"全省采供血机构演讲比赛等一系列无偿献血宣传招募活动
新疆生产建设兵团	"众志成城二十载,热血汇聚中华情" 组织《献血法》及相关知识培训,加大培训献血相关知识
广东	"为他人着想　捐献热血　分享生命"主题活动
山东	制作公益广告"血·缘"、微电影"生命速递"

地区	活动
安徽	"世界献血者日"暨《中华人民共和国献血法》实施 20 周年主题宣传 安徽省无偿献血公益之星和先进集体评选活动
天津	"津血同源　爱聚成海"大型公益跑活动
四川	充分发挥名人效应,将无偿献血作为第二季"李伯清话健康"散打评书主题之一 举办 2018 年四川省公务人员冬季无偿献血主题宣传活动 开展以"健康生活　快乐献血"为主题的健步走活动
云南	"无偿献血大爱无疆——你就是传奇 2018"征文活动 "818,熊猫侠,帮一帮"昆明稀有血型献血者品牌公益活动
上海	下发《关于开展纪念〈中华人民共和国献血法〉〈上海市献血条例〉实施二十周年系列活动的通知》 设计了纪念双法 20 周年手绘风格纪念海报 制作了上海市无偿献血 20 年专题片、出品了 2018 版无偿献血优秀志愿者故事集 编辑制作每月一期新民晚报社区版专刊《血液与生活》

为进一步做好关于无偿献血的宣传工作,营造"关心他人、大爱无疆"的无偿献血社会氛围,中国输血协会、湖北省演讲协会和武汉血液中心联合开展了"闪耀的红"全国血站汇报演讲活动。全国有 30 个省份的血液中心参加了此次活动。各位选手用他们澎湃的精神和感人的故事展示了全国血站工作者积极向上的精神风貌,向大家传递着无私献血的大爱精神,以进一步吸引和感召更多有社会责任感的群体和个人参与无偿献血,促进无偿献血事业的蓬勃发展。

三、无偿献血社会关注度不断提升

2018 年,我国无偿献血各级各类宣传活动进一步受到社会的关注,取得了良好的效果。广大群众用爱心践行了无私奉献的新时代献血精神,无偿献血热点事件精彩纷呈。2018 年 9 月 30 日,演员王凯拍摄无偿献血宣传片发布,其本人担任公益大使的新闻成为了 2018 年度网络血液舆情监测最大热点(见表 2-2)。无偿献血系列宣传活动如《献血法》实施 20 周年和 2018 世界献血者日纷纷登上热搜榜,全民关注无偿献血气氛日渐浓郁。2018 年血液安全热点关注度排名靠前的热点新闻见表 2-2。

表 2-2　2018 年血液安全热点新闻

序号	热点新闻
1	明星王凯任公益大使　无偿献血宣传片发布传播正能量(9 月 30 日)
2	陕西米脂学生遇袭　市民排队献血(4 月 28 日)
3	《献血法》实施 20 周年(10 月 1 日)
4	江西宜春"熊猫血"护士请假自驾　跨省数百公里献血(8 月 6 日)
5	安徽淮南警察献血表情走红网络(8 月 7 日)
6	2018 世界献血者日(6 月 14 日)
7	《献血法》实施 20 周年宣传片发布(6 月 8 日)
8	重磅! 成都积分入户细则出炉,献血等九大项可加分(3 月 12 日)

数据来源:全网监测和采集 2018 年全年网络舆情信息。

第二章

无偿献血促进

一、献血者表彰活动持续开展

我国不断健全无偿献血激励机制,每两年开展一次全国无偿献血表彰活动。2018 年 12 月 13 日,国家卫生健康委、中国红十字会总会、中央军委后勤保障部卫生局在北京联合召开《献血法》实施 20 周年暨 2016—2017 年度无偿献血表彰大会,表彰了一大批无偿献血工作先进单位和个人。其中,表彰无偿献血奉献奖 391 447 人,先进省 13 个,较上一届增长了 35.9%。

此外,为鼓励兢兢业业奋斗在血站一线的采血人员,国家卫生健康委、中国红十字会总会、中央军委后勤保障部卫生局决定对北京市红十字血液中心西单图书大厦采血组等共计 304 个采血班组予以通报表扬。20 年来,广大血站干部职工立足本职、敬畏生命,不断提高服务质量,强化血液质量安全体系建设,有力保障了无偿献血事业持续健康发展。他们开拓进取的精神和爱岗敬业的职业美德将激励更多血站干部职工积极主动地投身到献血事业中去。

此外,各省份还以《献血法》20 周年纪念活动为契机,开展各种评选活动。中国输血协会开展了"最美无偿献血者"评选,推选"最美采血班组"和"最美无偿献血屋"等,不仅提高了无偿献血者的满足感和使命感,也增强了百姓对无偿献血的认知感。

二、献血者激励机制推陈出新

随着《献血法》20 周年活动的开展,各省份采供血机构不断提升服务水平,优化服务流程。部分地区开展了"改善献血者献血体验"主题活动,着重优化服务流程,解决献血前排队等候问题。部分省份探索建立"互联网 +"无偿献血模式,实现"一站式"个性化服务,给献血者送去更多的关怀和更大的福利。部分血站在献血屋配置微波炉,为献血员准备多种甜点、饮品和纪念品。很多血站在采血室提供免费网络和电视服务。 献血后,除传统的电话回访、满意度调查、生日祝福、检测结果告知和血液去向告知外,不少血站还开展无偿献血者慰问活动,与献血者紧密互动亲如一家;与红十字会开展贫困献血者家庭救助活动;设立献血者助学基金等。部分省份将无偿献血工作纳入精神文明考核内容,启动"三免"政策(免费乘公交、免费进公园、免费挂号就医),极大地推动了广大群众的献血热忱,营造了良好的献血氛围(其他相关福利见表2-3)。

表2-3　无偿献血者其他相关福利

地区	福利
北京	献血者及亲属、团体献血单位职工同等条件下优先用血
福建	为献血标兵免费生化体检;赠送献血感谢卡;献血者健康指导;成立福建省无偿献血志愿者眼健康服务中心,为福建省无偿献血志愿者、献血服务志愿者提供眼健康综合服务
贵州	给予稀有血型献血者应急献血发放献血交通补助
河南	金奖获得者花会期间免费进公园;凭献血证看电影5折优惠;凭献血证驾校学习开车有优惠;与商家联系免费参加大型节日娱乐活动;发送节日祝福短信、开展节日慰问、设立助学基金等
湖南	全国奉献奖获得者免费体检;帮扶关爱慰问困难献血者
辽宁	志愿者和稀有血型爱心之家总结会;为获奖献血者送证书;献血屋献血关爱活动;为优秀献血者购买报纸等;献血者及亲属免费测血压
天津	为稀有血型献血者应急献血发放献血交通补助;为献血50次、100次的献血者发放无偿献血纪念奖牌;为优秀献血者购买报纸;通过微信为献血者进行血费直报
浙江	献血者住院关怀优先用血;慰问献血者,与红十字会开展贫困献血者家庭救助活动;血费医院直报、APP减免;为获得国家奉献奖金奖的献血者提供体检卡
山东	为献血者赠送人身意外伤害保险;实现血费网上减免,医院还血直报

数据来源:全国无偿献血促进调研表。

三、献血者权益保障不断提升

一直以来,由于血站与医疗机构信息不互通,"无偿献血,免费用血"的流程都是由医院先收取费用,献血者凭证到血站申请退费。2018年,部分地区积极探索献血者免交临床用血费用的直报方式,进一步提升了献血者的权益保障。解决了长期以来献血者及其直系亲属在用血过程中长期存在的垫付费用、手续繁杂、多次跑腿等痛点难点,更大限度地方便献血者。部分省份还制定了"无偿献血者异地用血费用减免管理办法"和"无偿献血者临床用血费用直接减免"等政策措施,大力推进血费直免,其用血费用根据规定在医疗机构实行直接减免,加大就医惠措施落实力度,简化减免程序,优先保障献血者及其配偶和直系亲属用血。以浙江省为例,杭州市实现省内血站与用血医疗机构无偿献血者信息互联互通,在医院开展用血费用"一站式"减免。陕西省推出《陕西省无偿献血者异地用血费用报销管理办法》和"无偿献血者临床用血费用直免"等政策,要求在2018年12月底前,省内所有二级医院必须开展血费直报工作。

　　与此同时,部分省份推动无偿献血奉献奖获得者享受优先就诊、优先住院、部分费用减免等便民惠民措施。

　　除了献血者可以享受免费用血和用血相关优惠政策外,越来越多的省份开始将临床血费纳入医保减免目录范畴(表2-4)。

表2-4　血费纳入医保减免目录的地区

地区	城市
北京	北京
天津	天津
上海	上海
重庆	重庆
安徽	蚌埠、亳州、滁州、淮北
甘肃	定西、嘉峪关、金昌、临夏州、陇南
贵州	安顺、黔西南、铜仁市、六盘水
河北	石家庄、秦皇岛、保定、廊坊、唐山、衡水、邢台、邯郸、沧州、张家口
河南	安阳、焦作、洛阳、濮阳、商丘、新乡、许昌、周口
湖北	武汉
湖南	长沙、常德、娄底、湘西、怀化、邵阳、湘潭、益阳、岳阳、株洲
吉林	吉林、延边、通化
江苏	南京、淮安、连云港、南通、泰州、宿迁、镇江
江西	抚州、吉安、南昌、九江、上饶、鹰潭、萍乡
新疆	乌鲁木齐、和田、伊犁
浙江	宁波、湖州、金华、丽水、衢州、绍兴、温州

续表

地区	城市
云南	昆明、文山州、红河州、昭通、大理、临沧、玉溪、保山、普洱、楚雄、德宏、西双版纳、怒江
四川	德阳、乐山、宜宾、成都、甘孜、阿坝、雅安、资阳、攀枝花、巴中、内江、凉山
海南	全省覆盖
广东	广州、深圳、佛山、茂名、韶关、东莞
广西	桂林、河池、来宾、崇左、梧州、北海、钦州

数据来源:全国无偿献血促进调研表。

第三章

无偿献血志愿服务

　　为持续推动无偿献血的持续发展,营造无偿献血良好的社会氛围,建立无偿献血的长效机制,各采供血机构非常重视无偿献血志愿者队伍建设。目前,全国大部分城市陆续建立起了多元化的无偿献血志愿者服务队,并发展为红十字会、志愿者联合会、狮子会及民间独立法人社团等多种组织形式。不少省份定期召开固定献血者联谊会,成立应急献血、稀有血型和单采血小板等多支志愿者小分队。部分省份建立"血站 + 社团"模式,一方面为志愿者组织提供办公场所和设备,另一方面开展动员活动、增进感情、与志愿者们保持深度合作。部分高校、社会团体和民间组织纷纷成立了无偿献血志愿工作者服务队,积极配合政府及相关部门,加强志愿服务组织管理,共享志愿者资源,并且定期培训。志愿者队伍在稳定中持续壮大,每名志愿者活跃在无偿献血宣传、招募、服务工作中,工作开展规范有序。例如,天津市探索建立招募团工作模式,开展集团式无偿献血。截至目前,有 20 余家单位组织献血。南京红十字会无偿献血志愿工作者服务队自成立以来注册志愿者已近万人,2018 年志愿服务总数达 2 546 人次,服务总时长 12 864.5 小时,创下历史新高。各省份成立志愿者小分队情况具体参见表 2-5。

表 2-5　各省份成立无偿献血志愿者队伍情况

地区	城市	总共在册志愿者人数	总共志愿者团队数量	总共志愿者服务站点数
安徽	安庆	80	3	5
	亳州	200	4	4
	池州	635	2	4

续表

地区	城市	总共在册志愿者人数	总共志愿者团队数量	总共志愿者服务站点数
安徽	六安	78	4	3
	马鞍山	276	3	6
	芜湖	550	3	6
	宿州	568	1	—
北京	北京	7 135	54	41
福建	福州	220	20	约50个(固定、郊县及高校)
	厦门	258	6	10
	龙岩	80	2	5
	宁德	63	1	1
	莆田	89	1	5
	泉州	235	4	16
	三明	3 036	1	—
甘肃	兰州	352	16	—
	定西	300	5	16
	嘉峪关	64	1	1
	金昌	50	2	2
	陇南	38	2	2
	平凉	2 000	15	1
	天水	162	1	9
	武威	61	1	3
贵州	贵阳	100	1	5
	安顺	377	1	8
	毕节	116	8	8
	黔西南	55	1	1
	铜仁	65	70	2
海南	海口	892	12	10
河北	石家庄	9 751	157	182

续表

地区	城市	总共在册志愿者人数	总共志愿者团队数量	总共志愿者服务站点数
河南	安阳	500	3	11
	鹤壁	315	3	1
	洛阳	330	1	12
	漯河	188	1	7
	南阳	346	9	18
	平顶山	1 635	12	10
	濮阳	580	1	10
	新乡	430	6	6
	信阳	804	6	2
	许昌	150	3	8
黑龙江	—	1 748	8	19
湖北	武汉	1 200	55	8(不含高校)
湖南	长沙	5 000	20	32
	常德	329	3	8
	娄底	176	1	8
	郴州	237	1	1
	衡阳	136	1	6
	怀化	286	4	4
	邵阳	220	1	1
	湘潭	5 264	30	10
	益阳	282	1	2
	岳阳	1 400	22	8
	株洲	695	1	15
吉林	吉林	70	1	2
	延边	126	1	1
	松原	458	1	2

续表

地区	城市	总共在册志愿者人数	总共志愿者团队数量	总共志愿者服务站点数
江苏	南京	1 158	1	—
	常州	1 050	1	16
	淮安	285	1	6
	连云港	2 800	11	105
	南通	1 028	1	7
	苏州	169	1	5
	泰州	391	4	4
	无锡	494	7	—
	宿迁	85	1	1
	徐州	2 218	9	32
	扬州	1 027	5	21
	镇江	91	1	8
江西	抚州	1 450	5	15
	吉安	249	7	17
	南昌	98	5	8
	九江	350	7	7
	宜春	385	2	—
	鹰潭	89	2	4
	萍乡	170	1	9
辽宁	—	2 750	44	57
上海	—	783	4 个支队 21 个分队	7
四川	成都	5 794	46	67
天津	—	2 538	2 334	28
云南	昆明	500	8	17

续表

地区	城市	总共在册志愿者人数	总共志愿者团队数量	总共志愿者服务站点数
浙江	宁波	445	12	19
	金华	138	1	2
	丽水	620	12	14
	衢州	225	1	2
	绍兴	424	5	7
	台州	400	9	—
	义乌	150	1	1
重庆	—	2 050	40	40

数据来源:全国无偿献血促进调研表。

　　经过 20 年的努力,如今,践行志愿精神,发展有经验的献血者参与到献血志愿服务中来,已成为无偿献血工作不可忽视的一支力量。我国大部分省份都建立起了"能献血、会宣讲、懂招募"的稳定的志愿无偿献血者队伍,形成了社会各界共同推动无偿献血活动发展的理想模式。

2018 年国家血液安全报告
China's Report on Blood Safety 2018

第三篇

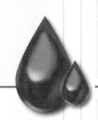

血站建设
与发展

截至 2018 年底，全国共设置血液中心 32 个，中心血站 321 个，中心血库 99 个，固定采血点 1 458 个，从业人员数量保持增长，学历层次不断提高，人员结构不断优化，血站基础设施持续改善，建筑面积增长较快，固定献血点和送血车数量保持增长，信息化水平进一步提高，血站已基本实现了本机构与献血点之间的联网。

第一章

从 业 人 员

一、人员数量保持增长

2018 年全国血站从业人员约 3.71 万人(图 3-1),东部的总数约 1.62 万人,占全部的 43.67%,其中广东、山东和江苏的从业人数分别排在全国前三位,均在 2 500 人以上;中部的总数为 1.08 万余人,占全部的 29.11%;西部的总数相对较少,12 个省(自治区、直辖市)的人数合计为 1.01 万余人,占全部的 27.22%,其中西藏人数最少,约 100 人,青海和宁夏次之,分别仅有 200 余人。与 2017 年相比,从业人员总数增加了约 500 人,增长 1.4%。东部和西部人数在增长,西部增长最多,增加了约 500 人,其中广西和贵州增加的人数靠前,分

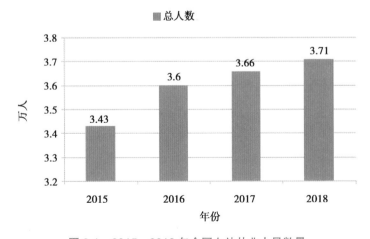

图 3-1　2015—2018 年全国血站从业人员数量

别为 200 和 100 余人;中部的人数减少了约 180 人,其中江西减少最多,约为 200 人。

二、学历层次不断提高

2018 年,全国血站的博士学历人员有 116 人,占学历人员总数的 0.32%,人员主要集中在东部和中部(除山西和安徽),合计有 79 人,占博士学历人员总数的 68.10%,西部的四川、重庆、云南和陕西合计引入了 37 人,其中陕西有 24 人,排名第一;硕士学历人员约有 1 300 人,占学历人员总数的 3.65%,东部的硕士学历人员最多,占硕士学历人员总人数的 56.16%,辽宁、山东和江苏的硕士学历人员均在 100 人以上,北京的硕士学历人员占比最高(9.20%),硕士学历人数最少的是西藏和海南(2 人和 3 人),硕士学历人员占比最低的是海南(1.12%);本科人数约为 18 500 人,占学历人员总数的 51.01%,人数排在前面的是河北、江苏、山东、河南和广东,均在 1 200 人以上,西藏最少(19 人);大专及大专以下学历的人数占比分别为 30.05% 和 14.97%(图 3-2)。与 2017 年相比,博士学历人员人数和占比在总体上没有变化,硕士学历人员占比增加了 0.14%,中部和西部的人数基本持平,东部的硕士学历人数增加 26 人,江苏增加最多(10 人),其次是吉林(9 人),广西减少最多(19 人),其次是湖南(9 人);本科学历占比增加了 2.84%,人数增加了约 700 人,东部增加 400 余人,其中河北增加最多(110 人),其次是江苏(103 人),江西和广西的本科学历人数减少最多(71 人和 142 人);大专及大专以下学历的人数和占比,总体呈现下降趋势。

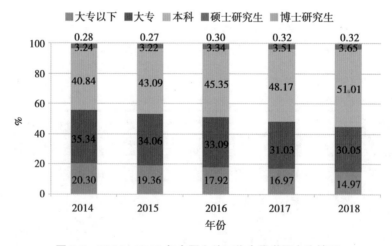

图 3-2　2014—2018 年全国血站工作人员学历占比情况

三、人员结构不断优化

2018 年,卫生技术人员约有 2.72 万人,占 73.44%。原卫生部印发的《血站基本标准》中规定血站卫生技术人员应占职工总数的 75% 以上,符合要求的省(自治区、直辖市)有 12 个,其中东部 3 个,分别是天津、上海和浙江,中部 5 个,分别是山西、安徽、江西、湖北和湖南,西部 4 个,分别是贵州、甘肃、青海和宁夏,比例最高的是湖北(80.40%)。比例低于 75% 的省(自治区、直辖市)有 19 个,最低的是西藏(55.88%)。卫生技术人员以注册护士为主,约有 1.38 万人,占比 50.89%,主要集中在东部,有 6 000 余人,其中江苏和广东排名前两位,西部的注册护士相对较少,约有 3 300 人,青海和宁夏分别为 50 人和 95 人,西藏仅有 7 人。注册护士比例最高的是湖南(62.63%),最低的是青海(27.78%)。检验人员约有 0.71 万人,占比 26.22%,东部约有 3 000 余人,江苏和广东最多,均为 500 余人,中部和西部的人数相当,青海和宁夏分别为 51 人和 75 人,西藏仅有 8 人。检验人员比例最高的是西藏(42.11%),最低的是北京(14.45%);执业(助理)医师和其他卫生人员分别约有 0.37 万人和 0.26 万人,占比见图 3-3。与 2017 年相比,卫生技术人员占比增长 2%。20 个省(自治区、直辖市)的卫生技术人员占比在增加,青海和甘肃增长最多,分别从 69.00% 和 65.70% 增加到 80.72% 和 75.92%,增长超过了 10%;11 个省(自治区、直辖市)的占比在减少,减少最多的是陕西,从 78.81% 减少到 73.67%,减少了 5.14%。此外,注册护士和检验人员的整体比例在增加,执业(助理)医师和其他卫生人员的比例在减少。

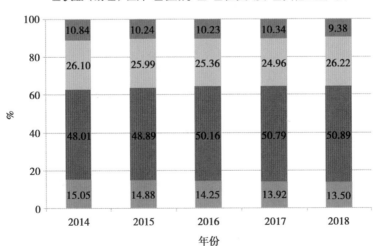

图 3-3　2014—2018 年全国血站工作人员构成情况

2018 年,血站行业专业技术职称从业人员约有 2.88 万人,占比 77.70%,高级职称、中级职称和初级职称占比分别为 12.56%、29.67% 和 57.77%(图 3-4)。东部的高级职称人数最多,约有 1 600 余人,占高级职称人数的 46.80%,中部和西部的人数基本持平,高级职称比例最高的是内蒙古(25.99%),最低的是安徽(3.76%),其次是海南(4.95%);东部的中级职称人数达到了约 4 000 人,占中级职称人数的 48.05%,中部的比例比西部高出 7%,中级职称比例最高的是天津(41.72%),最低的是新疆(19.15%),其次是宁夏(20.90%)。东部的初级职称人数约有 7 000 余人,占初级职称人数的 43.23%,中部和西部的人数基本相当,初级职称比例最高的是新疆(69.71%),最低的是天津(45.09%),其次是黑龙江(48.11%)。与 2017 年相比,具有职称的从业人员占比增加了 1.70%,中、高级职称占比均有增加,分别增加 0.38% 和 0.61%,初级职称比例从 58.76% 下降到 57.77%。东部的高级、中级和初级职称人数基本不变。中部的高级和中级职称人数均有增加,合计增加了约 100 人,初级职称人数略有减少。西部的高级、中级和初级职称人数均有增长,合计增长了约 300 余人。江苏的高级职称人数增加最多(36 人),安徽的中级职称人数增加最多(44 人),吉林的初级职称增加最多(92 人);河北的高级职称人数减少最多(10 人),广西的中级和初级职称人数减少最多,分别减少了 49 人和 190 人。

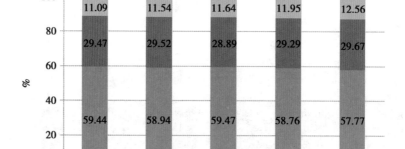

图 3-4 2014—2018 年全国血站工作人员职称占比情况

第二章

基 础 设 施

一、建筑面积持续增长

2018 年,全国血站占地和建筑面积分别约为 216 万 m^2 和 209 万 m^2(图 3-5)。东部、中部和西部的占地面积分别约为 80 万 m^2、70 万 m^2 和 60 万 m^2;6 个省(自治区、直辖市)的占地面积均在 10 万 m^2 以上,最大的是河南,达到了 17.70 万 m^2,最小的是西藏,仅有 0.52 万 m^2。东部的建筑面积约 92 万 m^2,中部的占地面积约 60 万 m^2,比西部多出约 3 万 m^2,建筑面积最大的是江苏(22.35 万 m^2),最小的是西藏(0.37 万 m^2)。与 2017 年相比,占地和建筑面积分

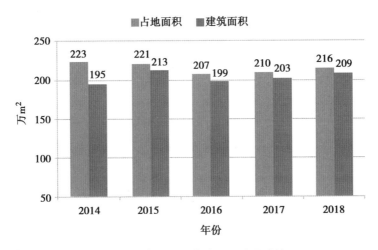

图 3-5 2014—2018 年全国血站用地情况

别增长 2.70% 和 2.90%。占地和建筑面积增加的省(自治区、直辖市)分别有 8 个和 10 个,减少的分别有 13 个和 12 个,江苏的占地和建筑面积增加最多,分别增加了 2.53 万 m² 和 3.12 万 m²,广西的占地和建筑面积减少最多,分别减少了 1.61 万 m² 和 3.23 万 m²。

二、基本建设不断完善

据不完全统计,2014—2018 年先后有 37 个血站选择了新址进行新建,涉及 17 个省(自治区、直辖市),新建前的占地面积为 12.51 万 m²,预计新建后的面积将达到 33.47 万 m²,增加 20.96 万 m²,增长 167.55%;先后有 15 个血站在原址进行了改建,涉及 10 个省(自治区、直辖市),改建前的占地面积为 7.18 万 m²,改建后的面积为 12.69 万 m²,增加了 5.51 万 m²,增长 76.74%;先后有 18 个血站已经完成了建设,涉及 7 个省(自治区、直辖市),建设前的占地面积为 7.14 万 m²,建设后的面积为 20.41 万 m²,增加 13.27 万 m²,增长 185.85%,具体情况见图 3-6。

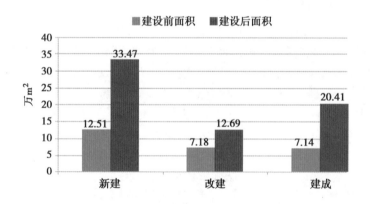

图 3-6　2014—2018 年全国血站建设情况

三、基础设施持续提高

固定献血点、流动采血车和送血车分别是反映血液采集能力和服务能力的重要指标。2018 年全国固定献血点、流动采血车和送血车分别为 1 458 个、1 583 台和 1 483 台(图 3-7)。固定献血点主要集中在东部(597 个),江苏和广东分别有 113 个和 112 个,位居前两位,海南只有 1 个,天津和北京各 2 个;中部的固定献血点有 461 个,河南和湖南排前 2 位,分别有 97 个和 92 个,吉林和黑龙江排在末尾,分别有 39 个和 30 个;西部有 400 个固定献血点,四川和重庆排名靠前,分别有 95 个和 56 个,青海 6 个,西藏没有固定献血点。东部的采血车最多,有711台,约占总数的45%,江苏、山东和广东的采血车数量排前三,都在110台以上,海南最少(7台),中部比西部多20台。东部的送血车最多,有598台,西部462台,中部423台。东部的广东送血车最多(117台),其次是江苏(99台),西部送血车最多的是四川(82台),中部最多的是河南(81台)。西藏、天津和宁夏的数量较少,分别仅有2台、8台和12台。与2017年相比,全国固定献血点增加78个,增长5.65%;流动采血车减少10台,下降0.63%;送血车增加12台,增长0.82%。固定献血点方面,东部的辽宁和浙江各减少1个,上海和海南没有变化,其余省(自治区、直辖市)均有增加,其中福建增加最多(23个),其次是山东(6个);中部的山西和河南没有变化,黑龙江和安徽分别减少2个和1个,其余增加,湖北增加最多(4个);西部的内蒙古和广西分别减少了2个和3个,贵州没有变化,西藏依然没有固定献血点,其余都在增加,云南增加最多(9个)。流动采血车方面,12个省(自治区、直辖市)的数量在增加,江苏增加最多(11台),11个省(自治区、直辖市)的数量在减少,湖北减少最多(12台)。20个省(自治区、直辖市)的送血车数量在增加,浙江增加最多(8台),7个省(自治区、直辖市)的送血车数量在减少,江西和广东减少最多,分别减少26台和22台。

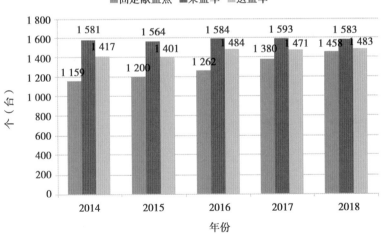

图3-7 2014—2018年全国固定献血点、采血车和送血车情况

第三章

信息化建设

一、血站联网功能日益完善

除山东、陕西、青海和西藏外,其余26个省(自治区、直辖市)均实现了血站的信息化管理。根据调研发现,血站已全部实现了本机构与献血点之间的联网;在血站之间联网方面,12个省(自治区、直辖市)实现辖区内的全部联网,7个省(自治区、直辖市)实现部分联网,还有7个省(自治区、直辖市)未联网;在血站与医院之间联网方面,4个省(自治区、直辖市)实现辖区内的全部联网,15个省(自治区、直辖市)实现部分联网,还有7个省(自治区、直辖市)未联网;在血站与省级卫生健康行政部门联网方面,14个省(自治区、直辖市)实现全部联网,4个省(自治区、直辖市)实现部分联网,还有8个省(自治区、直辖市)未联网。北京、上海、河北和江西全部实现了上述4种联网功能,占全部的15.38%。

表 3-1 2018 年血站信息化建设情况

功能	全部	部分	实现
血站间联网	12(46%)	7(27%)	7(27%)
血站与医院间联网	4(15%)	15(58%)	7(27%)
血站与省级卫生健康行政部门联网	14(54%)	4(15%)	8(31%)

二、信息管理模式不断创新

2018 年,我国部分地区在信息联网的基础上,不断创新工作模式。湖北省探索"互联网+"血液管理,建成集无偿献血者服务管理平台、临床用血保障平台、血液应急指挥平台、血液信息管理平台与无偿献血教育基地等为一体的综合管理平台。河北省通过对各地采供血量、千人口献血率、应急献血队伍建设等7大项、17个管理指标的实时分析,为全省整体血液管理工作的安排部署提供信息支持。广西全面建成全区采供血信息、血液库存动态预警监测、血液调剂、异地用血减免等血液管理应用系统,实现真正意义上的"从血管到血管"的全过程管理。浙江血液云平台已实现与省、市卫健委、全省血站(温州地区除外)、在杭州的省级医院、市级医院、市献管中心等的互联互通。同时,全省积极开展血液管理信息系统升级工作。上海临床用血一体化管理平台实现了全市血液管理机构、采供血机构和医院之间的互联互通、信息共享,以及江浙沪地区血液信息的互联互通。

2018 年国家血液安全报告

China's Report on Blood Safety 2018

第四篇

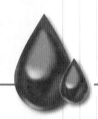

献血招募与
血液采集

第一章

献 血 模 式

为进一步优化我国无偿献血工作模式,提高血液安全水平,2018 年,我国全面取消互助献血。各地区通过强化无偿献血服务能力,加大团体献血等方式保证了临床用血供应的平稳过渡。一方面,加强无偿献血宣传与组织动员、增加采血网点,提升自愿无偿献血动员的能力。另一方面,强化团体献血的组织动员能力,有效解决献血淡季、血型偏型和突发事件应急血液保障等问题。目前,我国已逐步形成个人自愿无偿献血与团体自愿无偿献血协调发展的无偿献血模式。

2014—2018 年,我国总献血量和总献血人次持续创新高,团体无偿献血所占比例则从 20.7% 增长到 27.2%(图 4-1)。

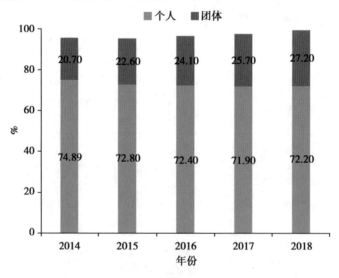

图 4-1 2014—2018 年个人和团体自愿无偿献血所占比例情况

2018 年,全国个人自愿无偿献血总人次为 1 067.6 万人次,比 2017 年增长 1.7%,其中,个人捐献全血 963.6 万人次,比 2017 年增长 0.7%,个人捐献血小板 104 万人次,比 2017 年增长 12.5%(表 4-1)。

表 4-1　2014—2018 年个人自愿无偿献血人次及增长情况

年份	献血 / 万人次	增长率 /%	献全血 / 万人次	增长率 /%	献血小板 / 万人次	增长率 /%
2014	970.8	—	897.3	—	73.5	—
2015	961.3	−1.0	881.9	−1.7	79.4	8.0
2016	1 013.1	5.4	927.6	5.2	85.5	7.7
2017	1 049.4	3.6	957.0	3.2	92.4	8.1
2018	1 067.6	1.7	963.6	0.7	104.0	12.5

2018 年,全国团体自愿无偿献血人次数为 402.7 万人次,比 2017 年增长 7.4%(表 4-2)。

表 4-2　2014—2018 年全国团体自愿无偿献血人次及增长情况

年份	献血 / 万人次	增长率 /%	献全血 / 万人次	增长率 /%	献血小板 / 万人次	增长率 /%
2014	268.3	—	265.8	—	2.5	—
2015	298.5	11.3	296.0	11.3	2.6	3.1
2016	337.2	13.0	334.5	13.0	2.7	4.8
2017	375.2	11.2	372.3	11.3	2.8	5.5
2018	402.7	7.4	399.1	7.2	3.6	25.8

2018 年,我国团体自愿无偿献血比例分布呈现地域性差异(图 4-2)。其中,上海市和浙江省的团体自愿无偿献血比例超过 45%,天津市、内蒙古自治区、湖北省和新疆生产建设兵团低于 15%。

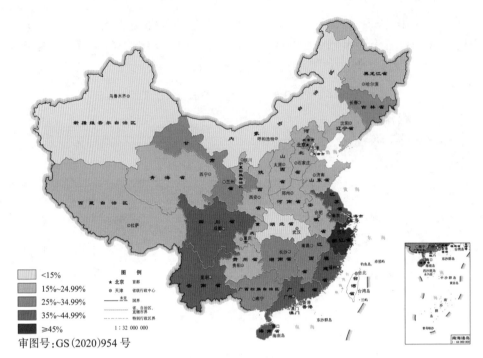

审图号：GS（2020）954 号

图 4-2 2018 年团体自愿无偿献血比例分布示意图
（注：本图数据不含我国港澳台地区）

献 血 人 群

我国无偿献血者的性别构成总体上呈现均衡发展,女性比例呈逐年上升趋势。男性、女性无偿献血者比例见图 4-3。

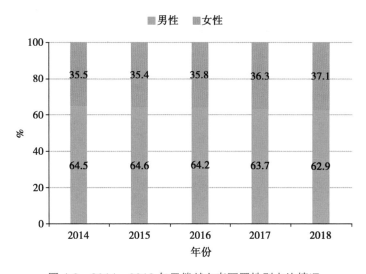

图 4-3　2014—2018 年无偿献血者不同性别占比情况

无偿献血者的年龄分布主要以 18~45 岁为主。2018 年,全国 18~45 岁无偿献血者所占比例接近 77.5%。2014—2018 年超过 55 周岁的无偿献血者接近 77 万人次,26~44 岁无偿献血者比例呈逐年下降趋势,45~55 岁无偿献血者比例呈逐年上升趋势(图 4-4)。

无偿献血者各学历人群以初中、高中、专科为主,本科学历献血者所占比

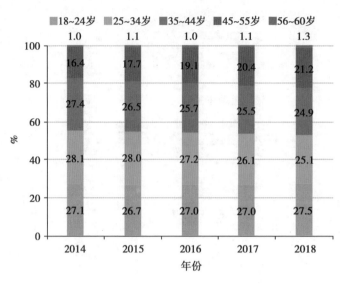

图 4-4　2014—2018 年无偿献血者不同年龄占比情况

例由 2014 年的 16.2% 提高到 2018 年的 19.8%，小学、初中、高中等低学历献血者比例呈逐年下降趋势（图 4-5）。

无偿献血者的职业涵盖了学生、职员、农民、工人、医务人员、公务员、教师、军人、不明（自由职业）等。2018 年高校学生献血人次占献血总人次比例为 16.3%，比 2017 年增长 0.7%，比例呈逐年上升趋势（图 4-6）。

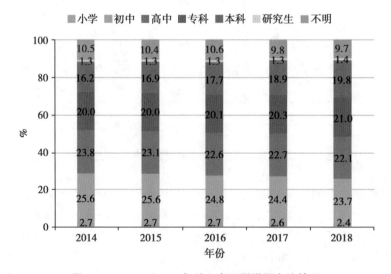

图 4-5　2014—2018 年献血者不同学历占比情况

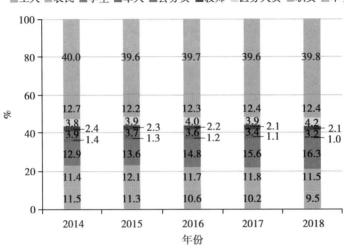

图 4-6 2014—2018 年无偿献血者不同职业占比情况

2018 年全国公务员、高校学生和医务人员在无偿献血工作中发挥了带头模范作用,献血人次占其职业人数的比例分别为 66.6/ 千人口、89.5/ 千人口和 55.5/ 千人口,远高于 11.1/ 千人口的全国献血率(图 4-7)。

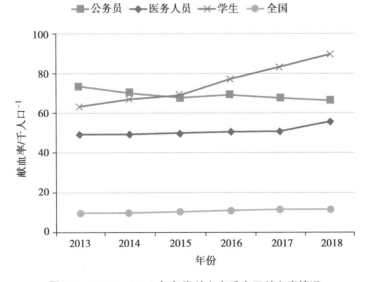

图 4-7 2014—2018 年各类献血者千人口献血率情况

第三章

血 液 采 集

千人口献血率是评价一个国家或地区血液保障水平的重要指标。2018年我国献血率达到 11.1/ 千人口, 其中, 北京市、上海市、江苏省、浙江省、河南省、陕西省、天津市等地的献血率超过 12.0/ 千人口, 西藏自治区等个别省份低于 6.0/ 千人口 (图 4-8)。在年度趋势上, 我国千人口献血率在 2014—2018 年

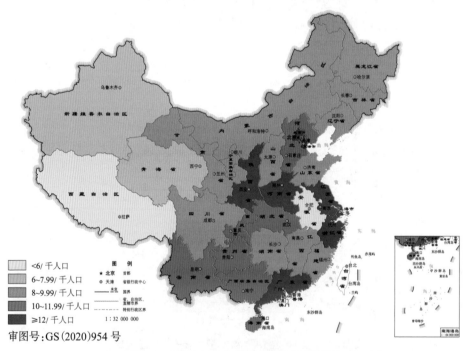

审图号: GS (2020)954 号

图 4-8　2018 年千人口献血率分布示意图

(注: 本图数据不含我国港澳台地区)

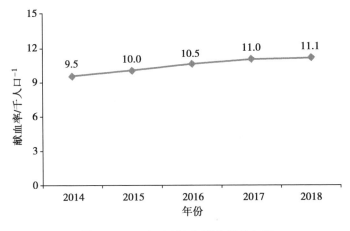

图 4-9　2014—2018 年千人口献血率

逐年上升,2018 年比 2017 年增长 2.9%(图 4-9)。

　　1998 年以来,我国无偿献血的献血量逐年攀升,保持了 20 年持续增长。2018 年在全面停止互助献血的背景下,我国无偿献血人次和献血量仍保持增长。2018 年采集血液 1 479 万人次,比 2017 年增长 1.4%。其中,采集全血 1 370 万人次,比 2017 年增长 0.9%;采集血小板 109 万人次,比 2017 年增长 6.8%(图 4-10)。

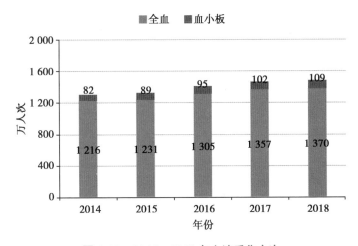

图 4-10　2014—2018 年血液采集人次

　　2014—2018 年,全国血液采集总量呈持续上升态势。2018 年采集全血 2 328 万 U,比 2017 年增长 0.4%;采集血小板 178 万治疗量,比 2017 年增长 10.9%(图 4-11)。

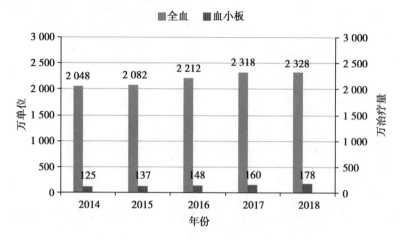

密性弃血工作,可以进一步保障血液安全,减少"窗口期"输血感染疾病的发生。2016 年以来,全国保密性弃血呈持续上升态势,2018 年全国血站保密性弃血为 5 297.4U,比 2017 年增长 53.2%(图 4-13)。

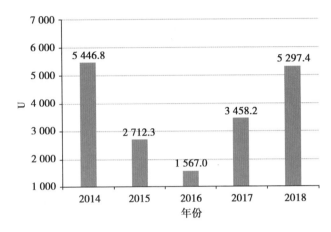

图 4-13　2014—2018 年保密性弃血量

2018 年国家血液安全报告
China's Report on Blood Safety 2018

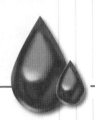

第五篇

血液检测和
质量保证

第一章

血站血液检测

一、献血前血液筛查

献血前血液筛查可以使部分不合格献血者放弃献血,有效减少血液报废和资源浪费,是进一步强化血液质量管理、保障血液质量的重要举措。目前,我国献血前血液筛查项目主要有血红蛋白(Hb)检测、丙氨酸氨基转移酶(ALT)、乙型肝炎表面抗原(HBsAg)、ABO血型、血细胞比容、血小板计数等内容。随着献血者健康征询和体格检查工作的不断完善,全国献血前血液筛查不合格率呈下降趋势(图5-1)。

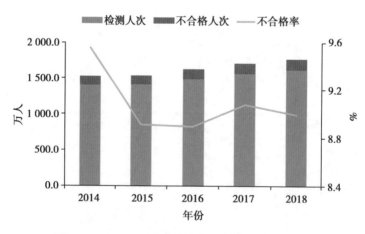

图 5-1　2014—2018 年献血前血液筛查不合格情况

2018 年,全国各地献血前血液筛查不合格率较高的地区主要是西藏自治区、青海省、宁夏回族自治区,其献血前快速筛查不合格率超过 14%,而湖南省、湖北省均低于 6%(图 5-2)。

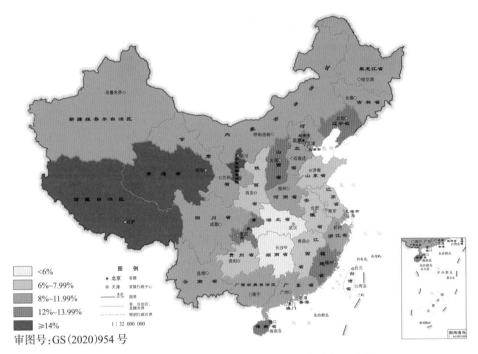

图 5-2　2018 年献血前血液筛查不合格率分布示意图
(注:本图数据不含我国港澳台地区)

2018 年,全国献血前血液筛查各项目中,HBsAg 检测不合格数比 2017 年减少了 6.3%,而 ALT 检测不合格数、Hb 检测不合格数比 2017 年分别增长了 3.8%、2.6%(图 5-3)。

2018 年,全国献血前血液筛查不合格的原因主要是 ALT,占比为 56.5%,比 2017 年增长 0.3%。HBsAg 不合格占比为 9.7%,比 2017 年减少 1%,Hb 不合格占比为 12.9%,比 2017 年减少 0.1%(图 5-4)。

从各项目不合格率的年度趋势上看,2014—2018 年 ALT 不合格率下降明显,HBsAg 不合格率呈下降趋势,Hb 不合格率略有上升(图 5-5)。

二、血液实验室检测

血站血液实验室检测主要针对输血相关传染病,包括 ALT、HBsAg、丙型肝炎病毒抗体(抗 HCV)、人类免疫缺陷病毒抗体(抗 HIV)、梅毒螺旋体抗体(抗

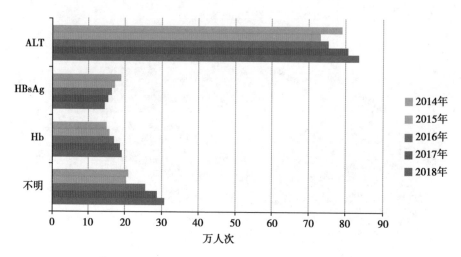

图 5-3　2014—2018 年献血前血液筛查各项目情况

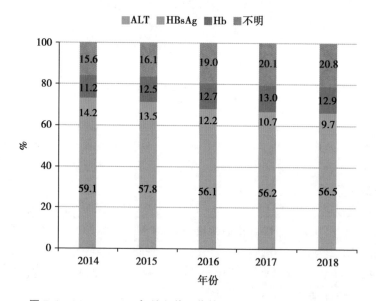

图 5-4　2014—2018 年献血前血液筛查不合格各项目占比情况

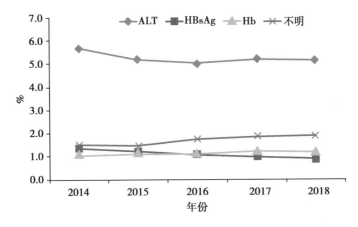

图 5-5 2014—2018 年献血前血液筛查各项目不合格率

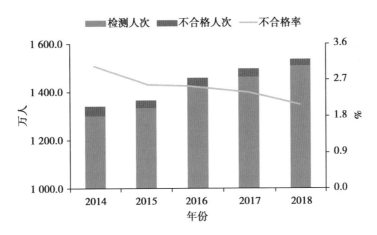

图 5-6 2014—2018 年血站血液实验室检测不合格情况

TP) 和核酸检测（NAT）。随着献血者健康检查和献血前检测的不断完善, 血液实验室检测不合格率呈逐年下降趋势（图 5-6）。

由于各地区传染病流行疫情差异, 各血站血液检测实验室采用的试剂灵敏度不同、灰区设置差异以及淘汰规则不同, 各地区的万人份血站血液实验室检测结果存在一定的差异。2018 年全国各省（自治区、直辖市）中, 西藏自治区的血站血液实验室检测不合格率最高（≥4%）（图 5-7）。

2018 年, 全国血站血液实验室检测不合格的首位原因是 ALT, 占比为 39.6%。其次是 HBsAg, 占比 19.1%（图 5-8）。

从各项目不合格率的年度趋势上看, ALT 不合格率呈明显下降趋势（图 5-9）。

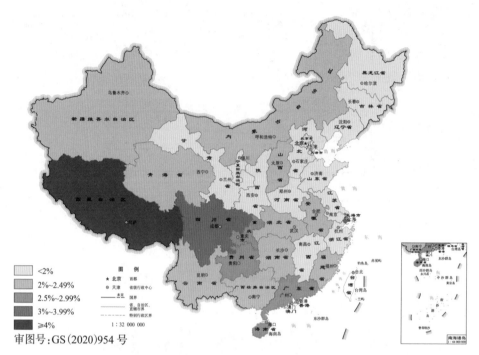

审图号:GS(2020)954 号

图 5-7　2018 年血站血液实验室检测不合格率分布示意图

(注:本图数据不含我国港澳台地区)

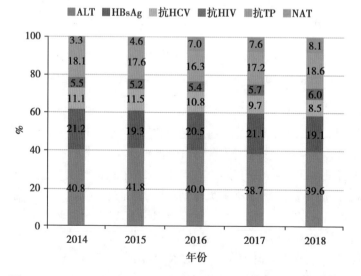

图 5-8　2014—2018 年血站血液实验室检测不合格各项目占比情况

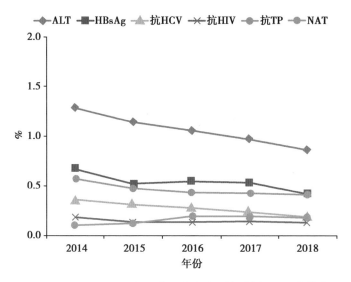

图 5-9　2014—2018 年血站血液实验室检测各项目不合格率

从 2016 年开始,广东、浙江和福建对全省献血者进行人类嗜 T 淋巴细胞病毒(HTLV)抗体监测,其他省按无偿献血人次的 10% 进行抽样监测。2018 年,福建省共监测 34.34 万人份,初筛阳性 269 例,确认 69 例,确认阳性率为 2.01/万。浙江省共监测 71.1 万人份,初筛阳性 109 例,未进行确认检测。广东省共监测 86.16 万人份,初筛阳性 277 例,确认阳性 13 例,确认阳性率 0.15/ 万。其他进行 10% 监测的省(自治区、直辖市)中有 24 个反馈了数据,监测总数为 104.9 万人份,确认阳性数 14 例,确认阳性率 0.13/ 万(表 5-1)。

表 5-1　2016—2018 年血站 HTLV 监测情况

年度	参加血站数 / 个	筛查样本总数 / 万份	初筛反应性率 / 万	确认阳性率 / 万
2016	138	250.4	4.51	0.61
2017	113	247.2	5.06	0.72
2018	94	296.5	4.06	0.55

第二章

室间质量评价

一、血液检测实验室室间质量评价

（一）实验室室间质量评价计划逐步完善

随着血液检测技术的发展和检测项目的增加,我国采供血机构实验室的室间质量评价体系经历了从无到有、由单一项目到多个项目全覆盖、上报方式从纸质信件到网络上报的转变,最终形成了目前较为完善的室间质量评价体系。目前国家卫生健康委临床检验中心(下称"临检中心")针对采供血机构实验室的室间质量评价包括4个质评计划的11个项目,基本覆盖了采供血机构常规检测工作,从而在保障血液安全中发挥作用。每个室间计划包含的项目,因血站、医院、试剂公司和单采血浆站/生物制品厂选择的质评计划有所不同(表5-2)。

表 5-2　室间质量评价计划基本情况

室间质量评价计划名称	开展检测项目	分类	参加单位		
			2016 年 /家	2017 年 /家	2018 年 /家
感染性疾病血液检测	ALT/HBsAg/anti-HCV/anti-HIV/anti-TP	血站检验科	376	366	355
		血站质控科、其他实验室	11	9	14
		单采血浆站、生物制品厂	40	40	60
血型	ABO 血型、Rh(D)血型	血站检验科	393	354	345
		医疗机构输血科、检验科	773	785	778
		第三方检验机构		43	65

续表

室间质量评价计划名称	开展检测项目	分类	参加单位		
			2016 年 / 家	2017 年 / 家	2018 年 / 家
病毒核酸检测	HBV DNA/HCV RNA/HIV RNA	血站检验科	217	333	307
		试剂生产厂商	9	6	6
HTLV 抗体检测	抗 HTLV	血站检验科	—	83	81
		生物制品公司	—	1	0
		第三方检验机构	—	2	1
		试剂生产厂商	—	3	2

（二）室间质量评价项目参评单位数趋于稳定

2018 年,有 429 家采供血机构实验室参加了感染性疾病血液检测质评计划,1 188 家(含医院)参加血型检测质评计划,313 家参加病毒核酸检测质评计划,84 家参加 HTLV 抗体检测质评计划。总体参加质评的采供血机构实验室数量趋于稳定(图 5-10)。

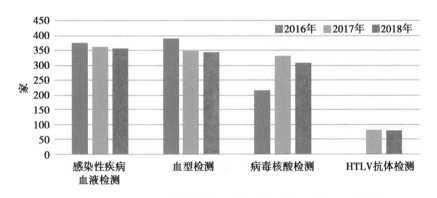

图 5-10　2016—2018 年临检中心室间质评参加采供血实验室数

（三）室间质量评价项目成绩保持稳定

感染性疾病血液检测质评计划:2018 年共进行三次感染性疾病血液检测室间质量评价,有 368 家血站的实验室(包括部分质控科)参加,整体符合率良好。按照三次质评均在 80 分以上即为合格的评价规则,有 350 家实验室血液检测室间质评成绩可判定为合格,合格率为 95.11%。

血型检测质评计划:2018 年血型质评项目改为一年两次,每次均进行 ABO 正反定型和 RhD 血型的检测,共有 371 家血站(含中心血库)参加血型检测的室间质量评价。ABO 血型正定型检测有 363 家实验室 2 次检测全部合格;ABO 血型反定型检测有 359 家实验室检测全部合格;RhD 血型有 364 家实验室全部合格;合计有 358 家实验室本年度室间质评成绩合格,合格率为 96.50%。

病毒核酸检测质评计划:2018 年共有 310 家血站实验室参加核酸检测的室间质量评价,其中全部正确的有 259 家,占全部血站实验室的 83.55%;两次质评得分在 80 分以上的有 304 家,占全部血站实验室的 98.06%。病毒核酸检测分为单人份检测和混合样本检测两种检测模式。有 65 家实验室使用单人份检测模式检测,274 家实验室使用混样检测模式检测。

HTLV 抗体检测质评计划:2018 年共有 78 家血站参加 HTLV 抗体检测的室间质量评价,75 家结果均为全部正确,合格率为 96.15%。

二、输血相容性检测室间质量评价

(一)室间质量评价项目参评单位数逐年增加

2018 年开展的质评项目包括:ABO 正定型、ABO 反定型、RhD 血型、抗体筛检、交叉配血五个检测项目,且均通过了中国合格评定国家认可委员会(CNAS)的 ISO/IEC17043 能力验证计划提供者认可准则的评审。参评单位主要包括医疗机构输血科、检验科、采供血机构实验室、试剂生产厂商以及部分部队医疗机构输血科、采供血机构,其数量从 2008 年的 200 余家增长到 2018 年的 2 144 家,包括:三级甲等医院 1 134 家、二级甲等医院 465 家、三级医院 276 家、二级医院 45 家、其他级别医院 109 家、血站 64 家、试剂生产厂商 9 家以及其他单位 42 家。2008—2014 年为参评单位的快速增长期,平均增幅为 39.15%,2015 年至今参评单位数量增长已经逐渐趋于平稳,平均增幅为 6.93%(图 5-11)。目前,参评单位已经覆盖 31 个省(自治区、直辖市),2015—2018 年全国参评单位具体分布情况详见图 5-12。

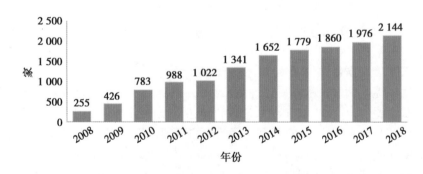

图 5-11　2008—2018 年输血相容性检测室间质量评价参评单位数量

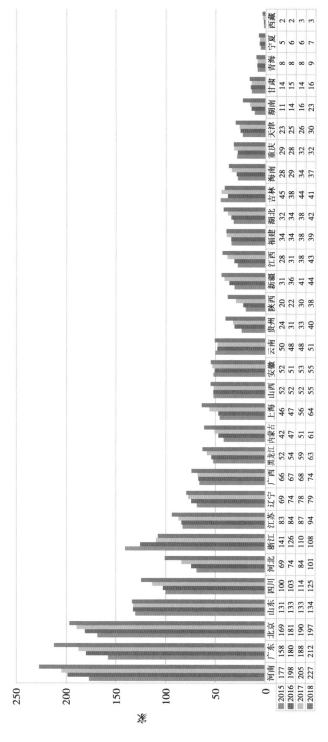

图 5-12　2015—2018 年全国省（自治区、直辖市）参评分布情况

	河南	广东	北京	山东	四川	河北	浙江	江苏	辽宁	广西	黑龙江	内蒙古	上海	山西	安徽	云南	贵州	陕西	新疆	江西	福建	湖北	吉林	海南	重庆	天津	湖南	甘肃	青海	宁夏	西藏
2015	177	180	169	131	100	69	141	83	69	66	52	42	46	52	52	50	24	20	31	28	34	32	45	28	29	23	11	14	8	5	2
2016	198	188	181	133	103	74	126	84	74	67	54	47	47	52	51	48	31	22	36	31	34	34	38	29	28	25	14	15	8	6	2
2017	205	212	190	133	114	84	110	87	78	68	59	51	56	52	53	48	33	30	41	38	38	38	44	34	32	26	16	14	8	6	3
2018	227	197	197	134	125	101	108	94	79	74	63	61	64	55	55	51	40	38	44	43	39	42	41	37	32	30	23	16	9	7	3

（二）室间质量评价项目成绩保持稳定

输血相容性检测室间质量评价项目每年度开展三个批次的质量评价工作,按照 ABO 正定型、ABO 反定型、RhD 血型、抗体筛检和交叉配血五个项目分别进行评价。2018 年,全国参评单位质评成绩为五个室间质评项目全部通过为合格,室间质评各检测项目质评成绩见图 5-13~ 图 5-17,2015—2018 年全国各省、直辖市、自治区参评单位的合格率见图 5-18。

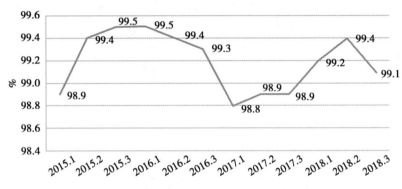

图 5-13 2015—2018 年 ABO 正定型检测项目质评成绩

注:2015.1 表示是 2015 年第一批次室间质评,其他依次类推(以下图同理)。

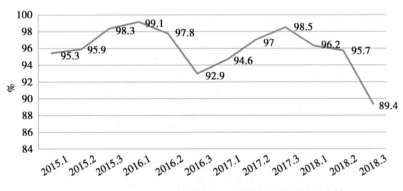

图 5-14 2015—2018 年 ABO 反定型检测项目质评成绩

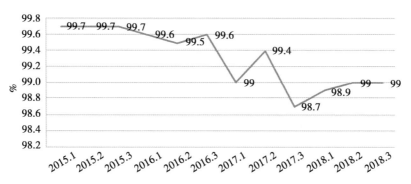

图 5-15　2015—2018 年 RhD 血型检测项目质评成绩

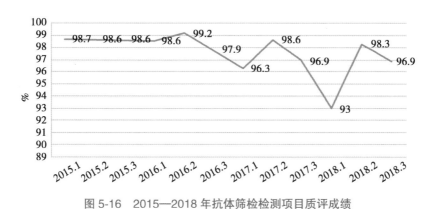

图 5-16　2015—2018 年抗体筛检检测项目质评成绩

图 5-17　2015—2018 年交叉配血检测项目质评成绩

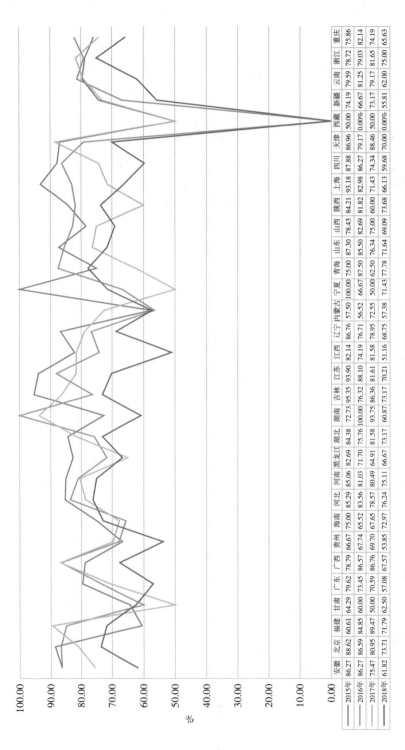

图 5-18 2015—2018 年全国各省（自治区、直辖市）参评单位全部五项合格率

第三章

质 量 保 证

为贯彻落实健康中国战略部署和国家关于血液管理的各项部署,各级卫生健康行政部门高度重视血液安全工作,国家卫生健康委按照"双随机、一公开"的工作要求,继续围绕政府领导的无偿献血工作长效机制的建立,临床用血和质量管理等方面开展 2018 年血液安全技术核查工作。各地在此基础上,以加强血液核酸检测和采供血全过程质量控制工作为重点,不断加强血液管理力度,推进信息化建设工作,创新工作模式,有力地保障了血液安全。

一、血液安全技术核查不断深入

国家卫生健康委一方面不断完善血站技术规程、标准和规范,指导各地加强人员培训和考核,强化血液管理信息系统建设,健全高危献血者屏蔽制度等;另一方面,为落实国务院"放管服"要求,强化血液安全和责任意识,2018年组织开展了面向 10 个省(自治区、直辖市)的血液安全技术核查工作,检查内容涵盖血液安全相关法律法规、质量管理规范以及技术操作规程,分别对血站、单采血浆站和医疗机构进行了深入的现场检查和指导交流。在昆明召开的全国单采血浆站质量管理会议,通报了全国单采血浆站质量管理工作会议精神和血液安全技术核查中发现的问题,提出整改要求。

二、血液安全执法监督层层落实

各省(自治区、直辖市)以提高血液安全和供应保障能力为重点,借助年度校验对血站和单采血浆站工作情况、换证期间执业情况进行校验和评审,确保业务工作及运营情况符合相关法律法规要求。同时,省、市、县三级卫生监督综合执法按照国家规定的监督检查频次(省 1、市 2、县 4),定期和不定期地对血站、医院和单采血浆站进行监督检查，日常监督与专项督查相结合，推进采供血系统依法和规范执业，完善采供血机构评价制度，针对血液安全重点环节要进行严格检查，及时发现血液安全隐患。将督导检查结果进行通报，并提出整改期限，督促各地对检查中发现的问题，举一反三，及时整改并提交整改报告。通过督导检查工作，进一步提高了血液管理工作质量，保证临床用血安全。

三、血液安全防控措施持续优化

一是各省（自治区、直辖市）定期开展内审和实验室室间质评，提升实验室检测能力。二是不断完善标准和质控体系。北京申请立项制定地方标准《北京市医疗机构临床用血技术规范》，修改制定《北京市医疗机构设置输血科审核验收实施细则》《北京市医疗机构输血科或血库质量控制指标》等质控管理文件。三是推进信息化建设。江苏搭建全省血液行政信息管理平台、全省异地用血联网减免平台、全省献血者屏蔽管理平台、全省血液调剂管理平台，甘肃建立了血液预警信息平台。四是开展培训。围绕采供血的各个环节，开展形式多样、内容丰富的管理培训班。五是开展血液产品质量抽检工作。安徽和广西每年定期对采供血机构所采集的血液／浆进行抽样，开展乙肝、丙肝、艾滋病、梅毒等四项输血相关病原体监测评价。六是引入不良记录积分管理。广西和四川分别建立了《广西采供血机构血液质量监测不良记录记分制度》，《四川省单采血浆机构不良执业行为记分管理办法》和《四川省医疗机构不良执业行为记分管理办法》，把采供血机构评审周期内的不良记录记分，作为技术评审扣分项目，督促采供血机构更加注重日常执业管理。

第六篇

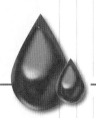

血液供应和
临床用血

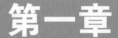

第一章

血液成分供应

成分输血是衡量一个国家、一个地区或者一家医院输血技术水平的重要指标之一。我国自 1998 年颁布《献血法》以来,输血医学事业不断进步,成分输血比例逐年递增。2018 年我国血站血液成分分离率达到 99.82%。

一、血液成分供应量逐年增加

目前,我国的临床供血主要有以下种类:全血、红细胞类成分、血小板类成分、血浆类成分。

全血:2018 年全国血站发出全血为 4.2 万 U,比 2017 年增长 36.1%(图 6-1)。

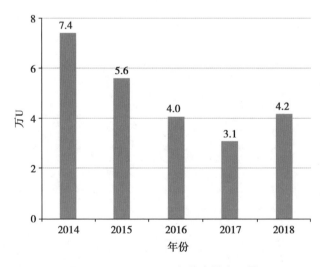

图 6-1　2014—2018 年临床供全血量

红细胞类成分:主要包括红细胞悬液、洗涤红细胞、冰冻解冻去甘油红细胞、去白红细胞和辐照红细胞等。2018 年全国血站供应红细胞类成分 2 260.7 万 U,比 2017 年增长 2.8%。其中,去白红细胞所占比例最大,为 66.2%,其次是红细胞悬液,为 29.2%(图 6-2)。

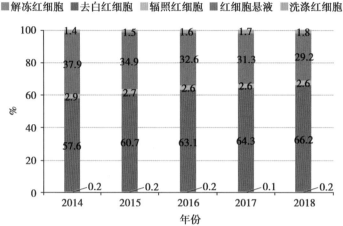

图 6-2　2014—2018 年临床供红细胞类成分各种类占比情况

血小板类成分:包括单采血小板和浓缩血小板。2014—2018 年单采血小板供应量大且逐年增加,2018 年全国血站发出单采血小板 177.9 万 U,比 2017 年增长 10.2%;浓缩血小板供应量较少,2018 年全国血站发出浓缩血小板 52.4 万 U,比 2017 年增长 34.1%(图 6-3)。

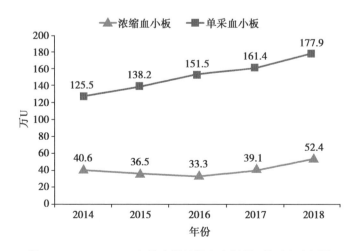

图 6-3　2014—2018 年临床供浓缩血小板量 / 单采血小板量

血浆类成分:主要包括新鲜冰冻血浆、冰冻血浆和病毒灭活血浆等。2018年全国血站发出血浆类成分达到 2 132.2 万 U,比 2017 年增加 12.4%(图 6-4)。

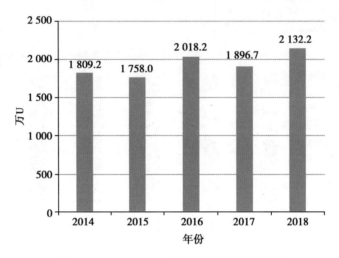

图 6-4 2014—2018 年临床供血浆类成分量

有形成分使用率是衡量血站血液综合利用和质量管理水平的指标之一。2016 年以来,全国有形成分利用率呈持续上升态势,2018 年我国有形成分利用率为 102.13%,比 2017 年增加 0.5%(图 6-5)。

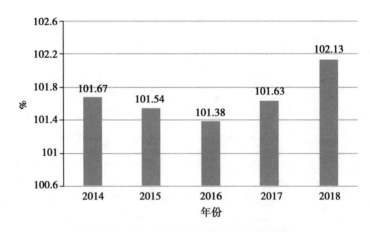

图 6-5 2014—2018 年有形成分利用率

二、血液调剂促进采供血平衡

2018年，我国各地区通过血液调剂进一步促进采供血平衡，有力地促进了血液保障，加强了库存管理（图6-6）。

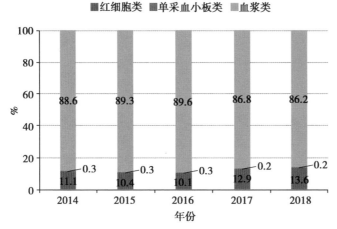

图6-6　2014—2018年血液实际库存各种类占比情况

近几年，我国各地区间调剂血液次数逐年增加，其中，主要为省内调剂（图6-7）。

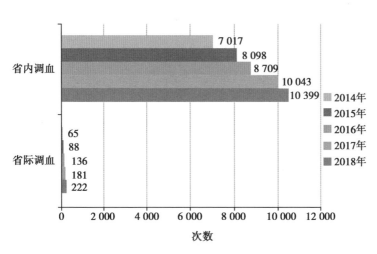

图6-7　2014—2018年调血频度

三、血液库存管理水平持续提高

血液报废分为检测报废和物理报废 2 种情况。血液检测报废指血液实验室检测不合格的血液报废和保密性弃血,而血液物理报废指因外观原因(乳糜血、血袋破损等)导致的血液报废和超过保质期的血液报废。血液物理报废是衡量血站管理水平的指标之一。

2018 年,全国血液物理报废量 151.2 万 U,比 2017 年下降了 1.2%;血液物理报废率 3.1%,比 2017 年减少 0.3%(图 6-8)。

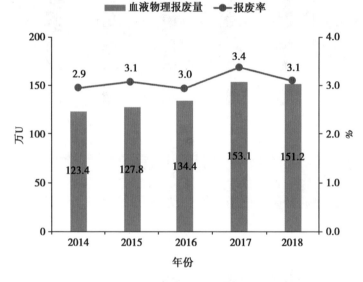

图 6-8　2014—2018 年血液物理报废情况

2018 年,全国血液物理报废主要是外观原因,占比为 96.5%,比 2017 年增加 0.4%(图 6-9)。

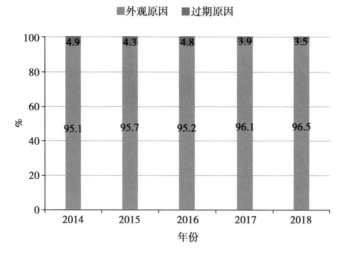

图 6-9　2014—2018 年血液物理报废各类型占比情况

第二章

临 床 用 血

　　2018 年,我国卫生健康事业发展统计公报显示,2018 年全国医疗卫生机构总诊疗人次比上年增加 1.3 亿人次,入院人数比上年增加 1 017 万人。在医疗服务量增加的情况下,全国的人均用血量为 3.3ml,较 2017 年增加了 0.1ml,全国每万人血小板用量为 13.1 治疗量,较 2017 年的 11.9 治疗量,增加了 1.2 治疗量。卫生健康行政部门以"提升依法治理、血液供应、血液安全和合理用血水平"为主线,多措并举,推动临床用血管理工作不断与时俱进,适应新的时代发展需求。

一、临床用血管理水平持续提高

(一) 临床用血管理制度、规范不断完善

　　国家卫生健康委《关于印发医疗质量安全核心制度要点的通知》(国卫医发〔2018〕8 号),将临床用血审核制度列为 18 项医疗质量安全核心制度之一,既强调了临床用血管理的重要性,又从全国层面对医疗机构核心制度的定义、内容、要求、操作流程和执行效果进行了统一;2018 年《全血和成分血使用》(WS/T 623—2108) 标准的颁布标志着我国临床用血水平跨入标准化的阶段,进一步规范了血液的临床应用。内蒙古、河北、河南、湖北、陕西、重庆、辽宁、青海、新疆、海南等省级卫生健康行政部门根据《医疗机构临床用血管理办法》《临床输血技术规范》等文件,制定或修订了本行政区域的医疗机构临床用血的管理办法、临床输血指南、质量安全手册、质量评价标准、管理指南、考核细则等管理制度,从制度建设上有效规范了辖区的临床用血管理。

(二) 医疗机构临床用血准入愈发严格

　　北京、吉林、宁夏、贵州等省(自治区、直辖市)通过严格对新申请临床用血的医疗机构或医疗机构新增设的输血科(血库)实行准入管理、对于已通过审

核的医疗机构进行校验或签订协议等形式,强化对医疗机构临床用血的规范化、责任化管理。

（三）医务人员合理用血意识不断强化

安徽、广西、湖南等省（自治区）以及新疆生产建设兵团通过公示、通报医疗机构的用血情况等管理手段,监督辖区内医疗机构加强临床用血管理,强化医务人员节约用血的意识。

二、临床用血质控水平不断加强

各省级临床用血质控中心通过积极开展各项工作,协助卫生健康行政部门不断加强医疗机构临床用血能力建设。截至 2018 年末,全国已有 30 个省级行政单位成立了省级的临床用血质控中心,其中天津和新疆生产建设兵团共 2 家省级临床用血质控中心在国家卫健委的考核中获得了优秀。各省（自治区、直辖市）通过不断推广临床合理用血的理念和经验,有效减少患者术中出血和输血不良反应的发生,保障患者的用血安全。

（一）临床输血质控体系建设逐步完善

截至 2018 年末,除江西、西藏两省（自治区）暂未成立省级临床用血质控中心外,其余各省级临床用血质控中心在各省（自治区、直辖市）卫生健康行政部门的领导下,不断完善省、市两级临床用血质控中心的建设。其中,福建省已完成全省 9 地市质控中心的建设,四川省更是逐步健全了全省的临床用血三级质控网络,截至 2018 年 7 月,已建立了 151 家县（区）级临床用血质控中心。

（二）临床用血常态化监管不断加强

各省级临床用血质控中心定期或不定期对辖区内医疗机构通过血液安全技术核查、临床用血督导检查、医疗机构临床用血调研等方式指导辖区医疗机构的合理安全用血。

（三）医疗机构输血人才培养逐渐强化

各省级临床用血质控中心通过举办政策、理论、技术技能等方面的培训交流以及省市优质医疗资源下基层等方式不断加强辖区内医疗机构输血人才培养。

三、临床用血新技术、新方法不断推广

各省级卫生健康行政部门积极引导、强化临床科室开展创伤小、出血少、成熟可靠的微创手术,实现外科手术用血最小化、临床用血精准化和质量效益最大化,减少手术用血需求及术中出血;积极推广回收式、储存式自体输血和血液替代治疗、患者血液管理（PBM）等血液保护技术,不仅有助于提高临床用血的安全性,还有效节约了血液资源。

根据国家卫生健康委 2018 年血液安全技术核查数据显示(以下核查调研

数据均未包含西藏、海南两地数据),通过不断推广血液保护新技术、血液管理新方法,各省(自治区、直辖市)在出院人次、住院患者手术例数呈增长趋势的背景下(图 6-10),核查调研的三级医院除血浆用量呈上升趋势外,其余各血液成分变化均较为平稳(图 6-11)。

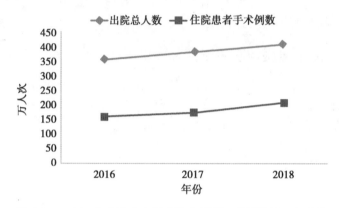

图 6-10   2018 年血液安全技术核查调研三级医院近 3 年出院
总人数及住院患者手术例数

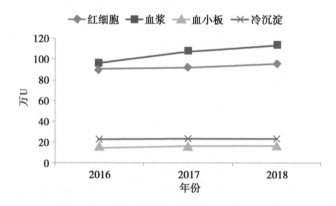

图 6-11   2018 年血液安全技术核查调研三级医院近 3 年各血液成分用量

核查调研的东部地区(包括北京、天津、河北、辽宁、上海、江苏、浙江、福建、山东、广东、海南等省份,下同)三级医院红细胞、血浆用量近乎持平,血小板略有上升,冷沉淀用量呈下降趋势,中部地区(包括山西、吉林、黑龙江、安徽、江西、河南、湖北、湖南等省份,下同)医院红细胞用量近乎持平,其余血液成分略有上升,西部地区(包括四川、重庆、贵州、云南、西藏、陕西、甘肃、青海、宁夏、新疆、广西、内蒙古等省份,下同)医院除血浆用量略有上升外,其他血液成分则基本持平(图 6-12~图 6-15)。

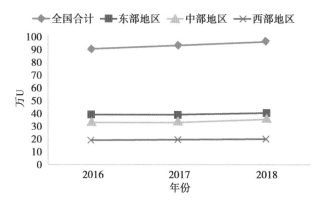

图 6-12　2018 年血液安全技术核查调研各地区三级医院近 3 年红细胞用量

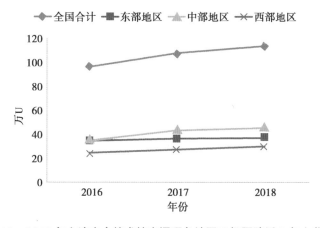

图 6-13　2018 年血液安全技术核查调研各地区三级医院近 3 年血浆用量

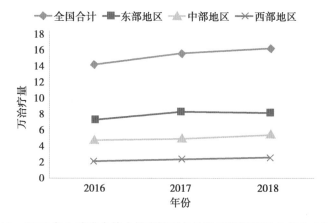

图 6-14　2018 年血液安全技术核查调研各地区三级医院近 3 年血小板用量

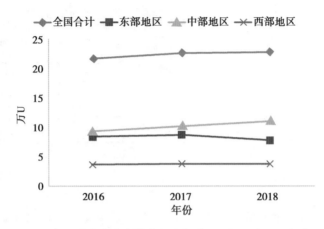

图 6-15　2018 年血液安全技术核查调研各地区三级医院近 3 年冷沉淀用量

医疗机构开展临床节约用血的各项技术,不仅可以降低临床不必要的大量备血及输血,还能降低临床用血的风险。例如中国医学科学院肿瘤医院(以下简称"肿瘤医院")开展了富血供肿瘤外科术前供血动脉栓塞术、临时性球囊阻断术、肿瘤出血介入栓塞止血治疗等介入技术。术前供血动脉栓塞术及临时性球囊阻断术可明显减少富血供肿瘤外科手术中的出血。如在肿瘤治疗的各手术科室广泛开展此项技术可降低临床不必要的大量备血及输血。对于急性大出血患者,血管造影可以准确地发现出血位置,行肿瘤出血介入栓塞止血治疗创伤小,疗效明确,可起到很好的止血效果。2018 年肿瘤医院介入治疗科共行肿瘤出血介入栓塞治疗 200 余例,止血效果显著,大大降低了临床用血量。

四、临床用血标准化水平持续提升

在各地卫生健康行政部门以及各省临床用血质控中心的推动下,医疗机构临床用血情况逐年向好。根据国家卫生健康委 2018 年血液安全技术核查数据显示,在出院患者、手术患者逐年增加的情况下,核查调研三级医院近 3 年总体的单次手术用血量、出院人均用血量、输血患者比例、输血患者人均用血量、手术台血小板用量均呈下降趋势,调研医院的临床用血愈加趋向合理(图 6-16~ 图 6-20)。

分地区来看,核查调研的东部、中部、西部地区三级医院单次手术用血量、出院人均用血量均呈下降趋势(图 6-21 和图 6-22);输血患者比例西部地区有所上涨,中部地区略有下降,东部地区降幅较为明显(图 6-23);输血患者人均用血量则是西部地区呈下降趋势,东部、中部地区有所波动(图 6-24);手术台均血小板用量总体呈下降态势,其中东部地区医院在 2017 年小幅上升后 2018 年降幅较为明显,中部地区则呈缓慢下降趋势,西部地区近 3 年几乎持平(图 6-25)。

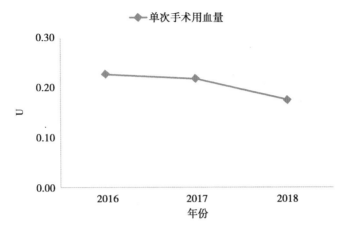

图 6-16　2018 年血液安全技术核查调研医院近 3 年单次手术用血量

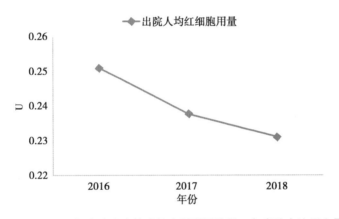

图 6-17　2018 年血液安全技术核查调研医院近 3 年出院人均用血量

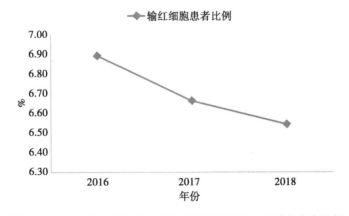

图 6-18　2018 年血液安全技术核查调研医院近 3 年输血患者比例

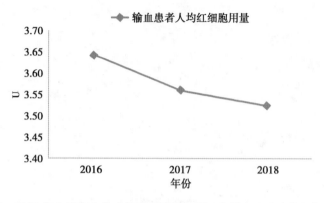

图 6-19　2018 年血液安全技术核查调研医院近 3 年输血患者人均红细胞用量

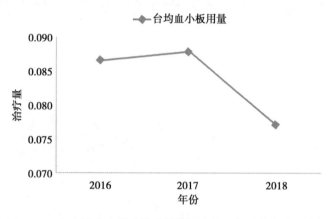

图 6-20　2018 年血液安全技术核查调研医院近 3 年手术台均血小板用量

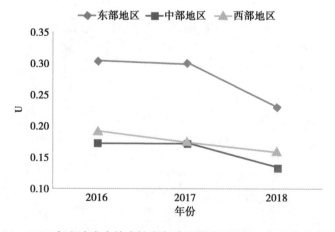

图 6-21　2018 年血液安全技术核查各地区调研医院近 3 年单次手术用血量

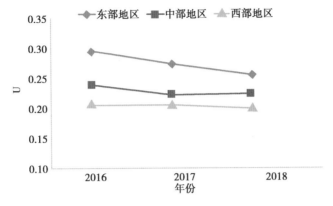

图 6-22 2018 年血液安全技术核查各地区调研医院近 3 年出院人均用血量

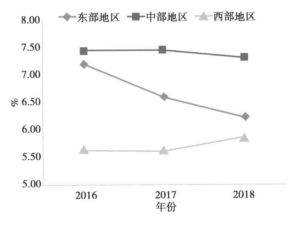

图 6-23 2018 年血液安全技术核查各地区调研医院近 3 年输血患者比例

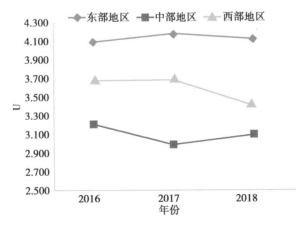

图 6-24 2018 年血液安全技术核查各地区调研医院近 3 年输血患者人均用血量

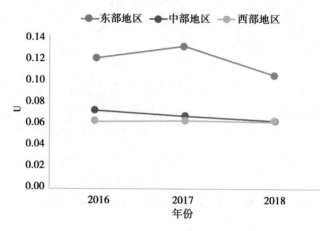

图 6-25　2018 年血液安全技术核查各地区调研医院近 3 年手术台均血小板用量

第七篇

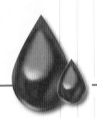

单采血浆站

一、浆站数量持续增加

2018 年,我国有 25 个地区设置了单采血浆站。其中,2018 年辽宁、云南、福建三个地区首次审批设置浆站,并开始执业。四川、广东和广西等地区的单采血浆站数量超过 20 家(图 7-1)。

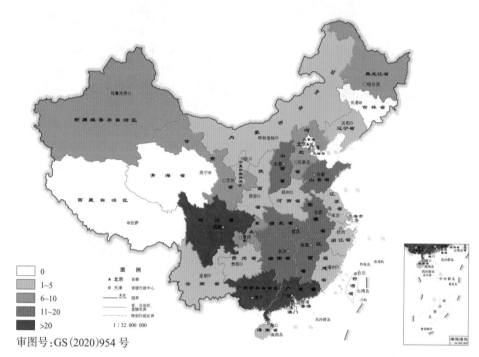

审图号:GS(2020)954 号

图 7-1　2018 年全国采浆区域分布示意图
(注:本图数据不含我国港澳台地区)

二、原料血浆采集量稳步上升

2018 年,我国采集原料血浆 8 343 吨,较上一年增长 8.1%(图 7-2)。原料血浆年采集量超过 100 吨的浆站有 5 家。

原料血浆采集量最大的地区是四川省,其次是广西壮族自治区和山东省(图 7-3)。

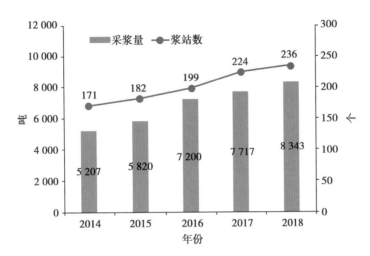

图 7-2 2014—2018 年全国单采血浆站数量和采浆量

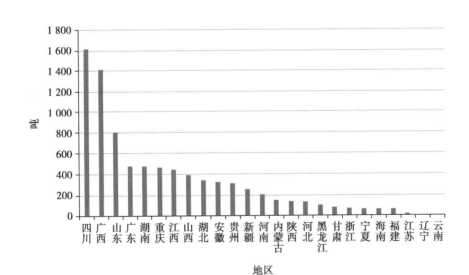

图 7-3 2018 年全国各地区血浆采集量情况

2018 年国家血液安全报告

China's Report on Blood Safety 2018

第八篇

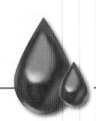

输血医学
科研与教育

第一章

输血医学科研

一、科技创新推动行业发展

经对全国 24 家省级血液中心、166 家中心血站、3 家医疗机构及 2 家科研机构的调查统计,2018 年,我国血液相关行业获批国家级科研项目(含国家自然科学基金)共计 13 项,经费共计 1 629 万元,主要集中在中国医学科学院输血研究所、军事医学研究院卫生勤务与血液研究所,研究方向主要为血细胞和输血传播疾病等。获批省部级科研项目共计 27 项,经费约计 230 万元,主要集中在中国医学科学院输血研究所、军事医学研究院卫生勤务与血液研究所、中国人民解放军总医院等,研究内容主要集中在血细胞、输血传播性疾病、临床输血和信息管理等领域(图 8-1)。

二、科技项目成果稳步增长

输血行业机构共获得省部级科技奖励共计 9 项(图 8-2),主要为经血传播病原体防控新技术及筛查策略的研究、输血不良反应发生发展的机制研究等。获批授权国家发明专利 23 项,实用新型专利 15 项(图 8-3),主要集中在血液运输装置、检测试剂及方法等领域。

三、科研论文水平不断提高

据不完全统计,2018 年输血行业单位为第一作者或第一通讯作者发表的研究性 SCI 论文共计 127 篇,影响因子总计达到 388 分。其中中国医学科学院输血研究所文章总数最多(27 篇)(图 8-4),发表在 *Hepatology* 上的论文为单篇影响因子最高(IF 14.079)。发表的论文内容涵盖了血液免疫学、传染病学、临床输血、材料化学、生物化学与分子生物学以及其他输血医学相关内容。这些 SCI 论文分别发表于约 50 种英文期刊/杂志,包括 *HLA*、*TRANSFUSION* 等在输血医学行业影响较大的专业期刊(图 8-5)。中文核心期刊共计发表 367 篇,非中文核心期刊共计发表 325 篇。

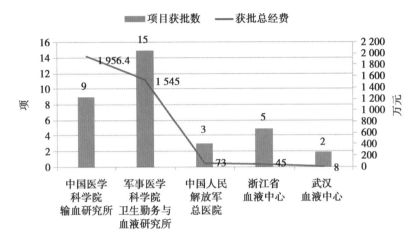

图 8-1　2018 年省部级以上项目获批总经费前五名单位

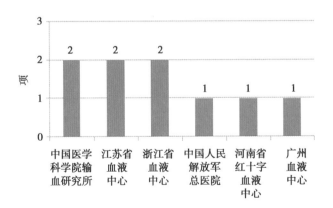

图 8-2　2018 年省厅级以上科技奖励获奖情况
（未包括省级协会授予的奖励）

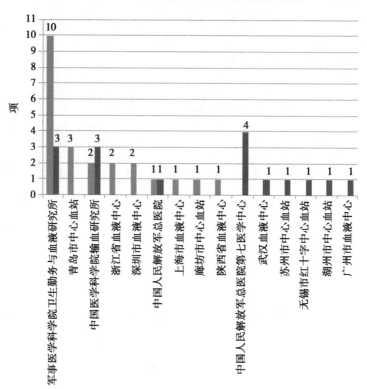

图 8-3　2018 年国家专利获批情况

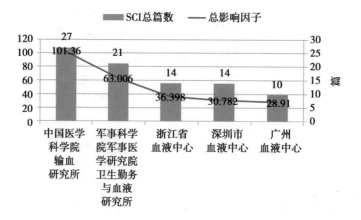

图 8-4　2018 年 SCI 文章发表总影响因子前 5 名单位

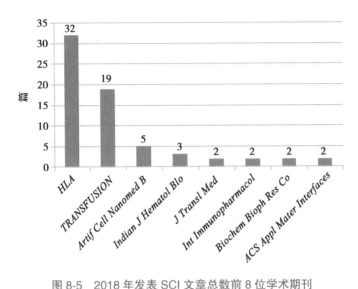

图 8-5 2018 年发表 SCI 文章总数前 8 位学术期刊

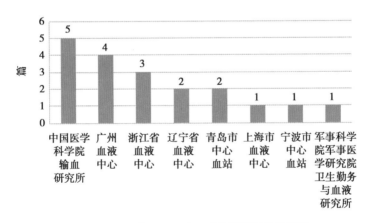

图 8-6 2018 年 *TRANSFUSION* 期刊发表情况

四、行业专著影响力不断提升

2018 年,输血行业出版了《2017 年度国家血液安全报告》《血液管理法制化历程》《临床输血技术指导手册》《血站消毒与感染管理》《血液成分的制备使用和质量保证指南》等 10 余部行业专著。由国家卫生健康委再次组织输血行业各领域专家编写的《2017 年度国家血液安全报告》,作为 2016 版的延续,对我国 2017 年采供血工作取得的成绩进行了总结和回顾。为庆祝《献血法》颁布实施 20 周年,由中国医学科学院、国家卫生健康委等专家共同撰写的《血液管理法制化历程》回顾了血液管理的法制化历程,总结了我国《献血法》实施以来血液安全工作所取得的成绩、分析了新时期血液安全工作面临的挑战,参考了国外部分国家血液管理的方法和路径,研究了我国血液管理法制化建设工作的思路和建议,提炼出血液管理的中国模式和中国经验,为我国下一步血液管理工作带来新的理论和方法。

第二章

输血医学教育

2018 年,举办各类省级、国家级继续教育培训班共计 130 余次,学员数量累计 20 000 余人次。其中,国家级继续教育培训班数量总体有所下降,省级继续教育培训班大幅增加,继续教育资源持续下沉。培训对象覆盖各级采供血机构、医疗机构、研究机构,培训内容涉及管理、招募、检测、质量控制等方面,为基层输血从业人员提供了大量学习培训机会,进一步提升行业整体业务水平(图 8-7~ 图 8-9)。

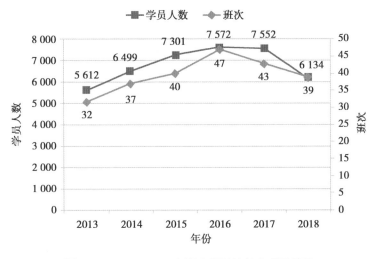

图 8-7　2013—2018 年国家级继续教育项目情况

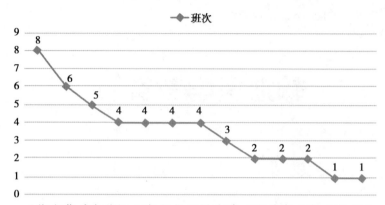

图 8-8　2018 年国家级继续教育项目地区分布情况

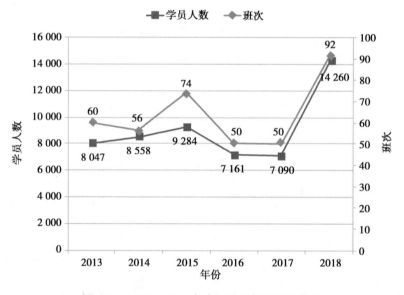

图 8-9　2013—2018 年省级继续教育项目情况

第三章

学术交流与国际合作

2018 年共计开展国内学术交流活动 50 余次,参会人数超 8 000 余人次。举办国际学术交流活动 1 次,参会人数约 30 人次。另外,共计 20 余人在各类国际学术会议中作报告发言,分享我国输血医学领域工作成果。

一、国际影响力不断提升

2017 年 12 月 11—14 日,APEC 血液安全网络质量工作组会议和第四届血液安全政策论坛在印度尼西亚首都雅加达举行,会议由 APEC 血液安全工作组主办,印度尼西亚国家卫生部承办。国家卫生健康委医政医管局相关负责人和行业有关专家受邀参加会议,成功向亚太区各经济体介绍了血液供应和安全保障的中国模式和中国经验,得到了与会大多数国家的认可。同时介绍了我国在无偿献血及血液安全保障工作中所取得的成绩和面临的挑战,特别是政策制定和实施上所取得的经验,并就血液质量管理问题进行了充分地交流和讨论。

2018 年 5 月 16—18 日,WHO 服务与安全部(SDS)和上海市血液中心 / WHO 输血合作中心共同举办的世界卫生组织合作中心以及血液与输血安全关键执行伙伴会议在上海召开。WHO 总部和 WHO 各地区办公室、国家代表处,输血领域的各行业协会和国际组织的相关负责人共 27 人出席了本次会议。会议的目的是协调 WHO 合作中心和重要执行伙伴在全球区域和国家层面支持 WHO 血液安全和供应充足性的工作。会议回顾了全球在血液安全体系建设中政策与策略等方面的信息与成功经验,各国在促进"墨尔本宣言——100% 无偿献血"上所作出的努力,以及如何获得更充足和安全的血液,并使血液的使用变得更为合理、公平。同时还探讨了进一步加强各国与中国政府、研究机构在血液和输血安全方面以及"一带一路"倡议下的合作机会。

2018 年 6 月 12—13 日,血浆蛋白 2018 年峰会(PPF2018)在美国首都华盛顿特区举行。会议由血浆蛋白治疗协会(Plasma Protein Therapeutics Association,PPTA)主办。来自美国、加拿大、英国、德国、印度、韩国、中国等国家的政府官员、研究专家、医生和患者代表,以及血液中心、血浆中心、血液制品企业、有关协会参加了会议。

2018 年 7 月 10—12 日,国际血液预警大会在英国曼彻斯特召开,由中国医学科学院医学健康和创新工程项目资助的输血不良反应发生机制研究团队受邀参加了会议,并在会议上介绍了我国在输血不良反应研究、血液安全管理上取得的进展,在血液安全预警工作中取得的成绩。

二、国际合作模式不断拓展

2018 年,我国部分采供血机构、医疗机构也纷纷开展国际交流与合作,合作领域不断深入,合作模式不断创新。辽宁省血液中心与法国国家输血研究所(INTS)就 OBI 的分子特征、发生机制与感染性开展研究合作。上海市血液中心与蒙古国家输血医学中心签署了"免疫血液学检测试验及脐带血库和造血干细胞库的相关试验的培训课程协议",为蒙古国家输血医学中心提供相关技能培训。成都市血液中心与斯坦福血液中心签订了合作框架协议。协议约定双方将在献血者招募、血液质量管理、预防经血传染疾病、HLA 检测、血小板抗原分型、红细胞免疫血清学等领域展开广泛、深度的合作研究,共同致力于提高血液安全和血液应用。云南昆明血液中心与老挝国家红十字会、国家输血中心签署了科研合作框架协议。

2018 年,我国采供血机构共计派出 50 人次前往美国、日本、加拿大、澳大利亚、以色列等地就输血医学、实验技术、血液管理等领域进行参观访问或中长期学习培训。同时,加拿大国家血液中心、美国斯坦福大学、法国国家输血研究所、澳大利亚国立血清学参比实验室等机构的 59 名专家来中国进行交流访问、培训讲学。

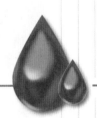

第九篇

不断发展的西藏
采供血事业

　　近年来,在党和国家的高度重视和大力扶持下,以对口支援形式为抓手,我国西藏自治区采供血工作取得重要进展。无偿献血氛围日益加强,全区采供血机构数及辐射范围不断扩大,血液供应总量及成分血供应比例大幅增长,自治区实现自主核酸检测,血液安全保障能力持续提升。

一、组团式援藏工作初见成效

　　自 2011 年原卫生部在拉萨召开"对口支援西藏采供血工作协调会暨支援西藏采供血工作签约仪式",特别是 2015 年"组团式"对口支援西藏采供血会议以来,各级政府对采供血行业的重视力度不断加强。在国家卫生健康委的统一部署下,确定 2017 年 7 月起,由江苏、安徽、陕西、广东、北京、上海、四川、重庆等 8 省份对口支援西藏地区,全面提升自治区采供血服务能力。

二、自治区政府重视力度不断加大

　　西藏自治区卫健委积极配合,一方面加大采供血基础建设投入,调剂 930 万元用于西藏自治区血液中心改扩建,落实 600 万元用于实验室改造及其他硬件设备更新。另一方面完善制度保障,修订出台《西藏自治区实施〈中华人民共和国献血法〉办法》,于 2016 年 1 月施行。

三、无偿献血宣传力度持续加强

　　在西藏自治区政府及有关部门的支持下,当地采供血机构开展了形式多样的宣传活动,不断提高公众对无偿献血的认知度和参与度。每年"6·14 世界无偿献血者日""世界红十字日"等宣传日,以及春节、藏历年等节日通过广播、电视、报刊等主流媒体及 QQ、微信等现代通信手段开展形式多样、内容丰富的无偿献血宣传活动。印制《西藏自治区实施〈中华人民共和国献血法〉办法》(藏汉双语)、《无偿献血知识手册》等科普知识宣传资料。在《西藏日报》《西藏商报》《拉萨晚报》等报刊刊登致无偿献血者感谢信。在出租车顶 LED、公交车、电影院、大型 LED 显示屏滚动播放无偿献血公益视频。西藏自治区血液中心推选西藏自治区歌舞团歌唱演员罗珍为西藏无偿献血形象大使,制作无偿献血微电影"重塑生命——西藏献血背后的那些事儿",荣获全国卫生健康系统优秀广播影视作品电影类三等奖。

四、采供血服务网络实现全覆盖

　　2015 年以前,西藏自治区内仅有 2 家血站;截至 2018 年,西藏自治区内血站总数达到 7 家(含筹建),增长 2.5 倍。西藏自治区下辖的 6 个地级市及 1 个地区均完成了采供血机构的设置和修建,实现了西藏自治区采供血全覆盖(表 9-1)。其中昌都市中心血站(筹建)用房面积 2 700m²,约是西藏自治区血液中心的 1.4 倍。自对口支援以来,全区落实对口支援资金共 855 万元,基础设施设备价值约 782 万元。截至 2018 年,西藏自治区血站用房总面积达到 7 000m² 以上,血站设置规划及基础建设取得重大进展。

表 9-1　西藏自治区血站基本情况

单位名称	成立时间	人员编制数 / 名	在编人员 / 名	实际在岗人员 / 名	用房面积 /m²
西藏自治区血液中心	2005 年	30	24	32	1 953
林芝市中心血站	2010 年	10	10	13	1 566
阿里地区中心血站	2015 年	10	6	9	—
日喀则市中心血站	2016 年	8	8	8	360
那曲市中心血站	2017 年	12	11	11	723
山南市中心血站	2017 年	10	10	10	—
昌都市中心血站	2018 年筹建	9	9	17	2 700

五、血液供应保障能力大幅提升

新建血站采血量逐年提升。阿里地区中心血站、那曲市中心血站、山南市中心血站随着采血工作的开展,采集全血总人次和采集全血总量逐年增加,2015—2018 年阿里地区中心血站全年采血总人次年均增长率达 19.8%。

血液供应总量大幅增长。西藏自治区建立了街头为主,团体为辅,应急为补的采供血保障机制。成立了由卫生系统干部职工、企事业单位、学校、驻军部队组成的无偿献血者应急队伍,同时建立了稀有血型献血者队伍,以确保满足临床用血需求。同时,自治区在国家"组团式"援藏的大力支持下,全区临床血液供应总量得到大幅提升。2016—2018 年,援藏累计调血 32 293.5U(含悬浮红细胞和血浆),占临床供应总量的 82%,极大缓解了当地血液需求。2018 年全自治区临床红细胞和血浆供应总量达 18 724U(含援助血液),较 2014 年增加 13 618.5U,年平均增长率为 38.38%(图 9-1)。随着供应能力的加强,全区血液供应服务范围不断扩大。截至 2018 年,西藏自治区血液供应医疗机构数为 71 家,较 2014 年增长了 195.83%。

六、血液制备技术水平显著提高

自对口援助以来,全区共有 38 批 400 人次赴对口支援省份学习血液管理、酶免检测、成分血制备等内容,支援省市专家 20 余人次驻藏以"师带徒"

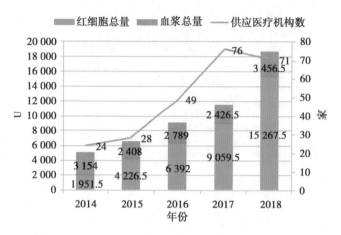

图 9-1　2014—2018 年西藏自治区临床血液供应总量

方式培养带教当地专技人才 290 人次,极大提升了当地采供血制备及管理水平。全自治区临床悬浮红细胞供应总量从 2014 年 1 951.5U 上升至 2018 年 15 267.5U(含援助血液),增长 6.8 倍。其中自治区血液中心于 2013 年正式开展成分血制备,成分血供应比例逐年上升(图 9-2),截至 2018 年,自治区血液中心临床全血供应比例仅为 1.64%。

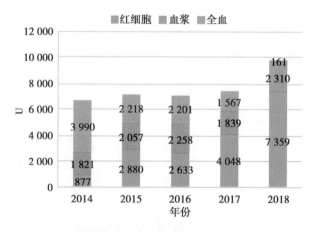

图 9-2　西藏自治区血液中心成分血供应情况

七、血液安全保障水平持续改善

西藏自治区所有血站均先后开展了经血传播病原体的酶免检测工作,有力保障了血液安全。在西藏自治区血液中心取得核酸检测资质之前,成都市血液中心帮助开展核酸集中化检测标本合计 7 354 份。西藏自治区血液中心于 2016 年 12 月完成核酸检测实验室改造和设施配备安装,2017 年完成人员培训,2018 年 1 月取得核酸检测资质,4 月开展血液核酸测,承担西藏自治区全区(除阿里地区外)血液核酸检测工作。林芝市中心血站于 2018 年 4 月起开展血液核酸检测与西藏自治区血液中心结果比对工作。截至 2018 年,西藏自治区基本完成了核酸检测全覆盖,血液安全保障水平有效提升。同时,西藏自治区加强了医疗机构用血资质审查。其中山南地区 2018 年在开展医疗机构用血资质审查中,取消了 10 家医疗机构的用血资质,进一步保障了临床用血安全。

2018 年国家血液安全报告

China's Report on Blood Safety 2018

第十篇

总结与展望

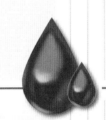

第一章

主 要 成 绩

2018年我国无偿献血总人次达到1 479万人次,全国献血总量达到2 506万U,献血率达到11.1/千人口。2018年无偿献血总人次和采血量较去年增长1.4%和1.1%。我国已基本形成了体系完善、管理科学、保障有力、使用合理的无偿献血工作格局,各项工作实现跨越式发展。

一、血液管理法制建设不断完善,血液安全保障能力不断提高

全国各地、各部门认真贯彻落实《献血法》,依法加强组织领导,完善无偿献血工作机制。逐步形成国家《献血法》、省级“实施《献血法》条例”,地市“落实《献血法》办法”的三级法制化体系建设。各级卫生健康、财政、发展改革、宣传等部门协调联动,尽职履责,推进区域内无偿献血工作。随着法制体系的不断完善,行业标准制定的不断科学,血液安全得到了有力的保障。

二、无偿献血社会氛围日益活跃,无偿献血获奖人数显著增加

各地积极开展无偿献血宣传招募工作,营造良好的社会氛围。在无偿献血公益宣传日,由国家到各省(自治区、直辖市)组织开展一系列形式多样、内容丰富的公益宣传活动,形成了积极向上的无偿献血舆论氛围。2018年12月12日,国家卫生健康委员会、中国红十字会总会和中央军委后勤保障部卫生局联合发布《关于表彰2016—2017年度无偿献血奉献奖金奖等奖项获奖者的决定》。本届表彰中,无偿献血奉献奖人数超过39万,较上一届增长了35.9%,获奖人数显著增加。持续开展的献血者表彰活动和创新的激励机制,让无偿献血工作得到全社会的广泛理解和支持,越来越多的公众加入到无偿献血者

队伍中来,无偿献血事业发展呈现出健康、可持续的良好态势。

三、血液采供服务网络不断延伸,边远地区血液安全持续改善

为保障我国血液供应,各地按照血站设置规划要求,合理配置血站建设。坚持以献血者和患者为中心,不断完善服务设施,增强服务意识,优化服务流程,健全完善血站服务体系。截至 2018 年底,西藏地区所有血站全部正式执业,全国 452 家血站全部投入运营。血站基础条件、建筑设施、设备仪器持续改善,从业人员总数逐步增多、结构不断优化,高学历从业人员和卫生技术人员占比持续增加。2018 年 4 月,西藏自治区血液中心独立开展血液核酸检测。至此,全国 31 个省(自治区、直辖市)及新疆生产建设兵团均具备核酸检测能力,我国血液安全保障能力迈上新台阶。

四、血液质量管理体系不断完善,血液检测质控水平持续提升

我国建立了覆盖采供血全过程的血液质量管理体系,形成了较为完善的采供血机构实验室室间质量评价体系和临床输血相容性检测室间质量评价体系。采供血机构实验室室间质量评价体系基本覆盖了采供血机构常规检测工作,2018 年各项评价项目成绩保持稳定。临床输血相容性检测室间质量评价体系参评单位已覆盖全国的 31 个省(自治区、直辖市),2018 年全国参评单位五项室间质评项目质评成绩全部通过,在保障血液安全中发挥了重要作用。

五、血液安全执法监督层层落实,血液安全防控措施持续优化

为强化血液安全意识,落实血液安全责任,保障临床用血供应与安全,国家卫生健康委抽查了 10 个省(自治区、直辖市)的部分采供血机构和医院,开展血液安全技术核查工作。同时,各省(自治区、直辖市)卫生健康行政部门和卫生监督执法部门按照国家相关规定,定期和不定期地对采供血机构和医院进行监督检查。形成了由上至下、覆盖全面、标准统一的执法监督体系,保障了采供血系统依法依规执业,完善了采供血机构评价制度,及时对发现的安全隐患进行整改,进一步保障了献血者和用血者的安全。

六、临床用血管理水平不断提高,新技术新方法不断推广

国家及各省(自治区、直辖市)卫生健康行政部门从制度、行业规范、新机构准入等渠道不断加强临床用血管理。在各级卫生健康行政部门的指导下,各级临床输血质量控制中心体系建设不断完善,各级临床输血质控中心通过临床合理用血评价、监督、管理和考核等质量管理手段以及新技术推广、人员

培训等工作为抓手,一方面不断加强临床安全用血,另一方面在住院量和手术量持续增长的情况下,手术台均用血量、出院人均用血量、输血患者比例、输血患者人均用血量、手术台均血小板用量等临床用血相关指标均呈下降趋势,临床用血更为合理。

第二章

面临的挑战

一、血液供应依然面临挑战

近年来,随着健康中国战略的不断推进,人均期望寿命持续增长,进一步加重人口老龄化。二孩政策全面实施使得大龄产妇数量增加,医疗保障水平提高使得医疗服务量持续增长,这些都对血液的供应提出了更新和更高的要求。目前,我国血液供应仍然处于"紧平衡"状态。千人口献血率等指标较发达国家仍有差距,血液供需矛盾依然面临挑战。

二、边远地区自身采供血能力有待提高

在国家各级政府的高度重视和大力扶持下,边疆地区采供血各项工作持续发展。但因边疆地区采供血工作起步晚,无偿献血社会氛围仍有待提高,保障机制仍需改进。同时受传统观念的影响,少数民族公民主动无偿献血积极性不高,无偿献血人群主要以汉族人员为主。此外,边疆地区采供血机构一直面临卫生技术人才数量不足,人才队伍整体素质不高及人才流失等问题,人才问题仍是制约边疆地区采供血能力发展的关键因素之一。因此,在提升边疆地区自身血液供应和保障能力方面,仍面临着挑战。

三、血液安全风险仍然存在

2018 年,我国南方部分地区发生登革热疫情,登革热也是经输血传播的病原体,提示在新发、再发经血传播病原体防控上,我国依然面积挑战。目前,在经血传播病原体筛查上,我国较欧美、日本等地区仍有差距。地方性、时限性输血相关传染病标志物检测尚缺乏大样本多中心流行病学数据。

第三章

展 望

一、探索无偿献血的长效机制

无偿献血是一项社会性很强的医疗卫生事业,各级地方政府需要进一步健全"政府领导、部门合作、全社会参与"的无偿献血长效工作机制,切实担负起保障和改善民生的重要职责。加大财政投入力度,完善血站基础设施建设,确保血站服务体系与卫生健康事业发展相适应。建立适宜血站工作人员发展的薪酬制度,加强专业技术人才队伍的培养和发展。同时创新机制,探索无偿献血宣传招募的激励措施,形成弘扬无偿献血价值理念的社会氛围,不断壮大献血者队伍。

二、优化采供血体系建设

目前,我国多数地区血站规模小,功能不全,人才留不住,运行成本高。参考发达国家的经验和世界卫生组织的建议,积极探索"分散采集、统一制备、集中检测"的发展模式。通过成熟的固定采血点和新设置的流动采血点,不断提升服务水平和服务能力,进一步保障血液供应。按区域统一设置血液成分制备、按省份开展血液集中化检测可以进一步强化实验室设施,保证人员配备,降低运行成本,提高血液质量。

三、提高采供血精细化管理能力水平

建立采供血机构全面质量管理,加快推进血液管理信息全国联网,完善覆盖采供血和临床用血全过程的血液管理信息化建设,从而加强血液的标准化和精细化管理。探索"优质、高效、便捷"的血站服务模式,合理规划血站业务区域布局,优化业务流程,提高服务满意度。提高血站工作人员的服务意识、规范服务行为、改进服务质量,提高献血者的获得感,进一步保证血液质量和安全。

四、推进临床合理用血标准化管理

进一步推进患者血液管理(PBM)工作,推进临床合理用血的标准化管理。开展临床用血评价,进一步提高科学、合理用血水平。不断健全临床用血监督、管理和通报制度,推广合理用血新技术,减少不必要输血,实现临床用血精准化和质量效益最大化,节约血液资源。

五、建立血液安全风险预警机制

逐步推广输血不良反应监测工作,建立我国血液安全预警机制,提前预防和阻断可能发生的血液安全风险。建立统一的输血安全监测体系和血液安全预警制度,完善输血不良反应上报系统,提高输血不良反应的诊断、分类、分级、治疗及预防能力和水平,降低输血不良反应的发生,提高患者安全。

附　录

附表 1　2018 年千人口献血率汇总表

序号	地区	/千人口 $^{-1}$	比 2017 年增长	
			/千人口 $^{-1}$	增长率 /%
1	北京	16.3	−1.0	−5.8
2	天津	12.2	0.6	5.5
3	河北	10.6	0.4	4.1
4	山西	9.9	0.6	6.7
5	内蒙古	8.7	0.4	4.3
6	辽宁	9.8	−0.2	−2.1
7	吉林	9.9	0.4	3.7
8	黑龙江	9.9	0.3	2.6
9	上海	14.8	0.0	−0.1
10	江苏	13.0	0.6	4.4
11	浙江	12.5	0.4	3.4
12	安徽	7.8	0.1	0.8
13	福建	8.7	0.0	−0.1
14	江西	8.6	0.5	6.3
15	山东	10.3	0.2	2.0
16	河南	12.3	0.6	5.2
17	湖北	11.6	0.3	2.9
18	湖南	8.6	0.1	1.0
19	广东	12.0	−0.1	−1.0
20	广西	11.2	0.2	1.5

续表

序号	地区	/千人口 $^{-1}$	比 2017 年增长	
			/千人口 $^{-1}$	增长率 /%
21	海南	11.3	0.2	2.0
22	重庆	11.1	0.1	0.5
23	四川	9.3	0.3	3.5
24	贵州	10.2	0.4	4.4
25	云南	10.1	0.7	7.3
26	西藏	0.5	−0.5	−49.9
27	陕西	12.3	0.3	2.7
28	甘肃	8.1	0.0	−0.4
29	青海	7.6	−0.2	−2.4
30	宁夏	9.4	−0.4	−4.0
31	新疆	6.3	−0.2	−2.7
32	兵团	5.8	−0.6	−10.0

附表 2　2018 年血液采集情况汇总表

序号	地区	全血			血小板		
		/万 U	比 2017 年增长		/万治疗量	比 2017 年增长	
			/万 U	增长率 /%		/万治疗量	增长率 /%
1	北京	50.6	−3.6	−6.6	8.8	−1.6	−15.5
2	天津	28.9	1.4	5.0	5.5	0.4	8.8
3	河北	136.5	4.9	3.7	10.8	0.7	7.4
4	山西	65.4	3.5	5.6	4.0	1.1	36.8
5	内蒙古	36.4	1.4	3.9	2.1	0.2	10.0
6	辽宁	70.6	−1.6	−2.3	5.3	−0.1	−1.0
7	吉林	42.4	1.7	4.1	2.8	0.2	8.5
8	黑龙江	63.7	1.7	2.8	3.7	0.1	3.6

续表

序号	地区	全血			血小板		
		/万U	比2017年增长		/万治疗量	比2017年增长	
			/万U	增长率/%		/万治疗量	增长率/%
9	上海	45.7	−0.8	−1.6	4.5	0.4	8.5
10	江苏	152.8	7.6	5.2	16.4	1.4	9.4
11	浙江	100.3	4.8	5.0	9.7	1.0	12.0
12	安徽	76.4	0.3	0.3	3.7	0.4	12.8
13	福建	52.9	0.5	1.0	3.7	0.2	5.4
14	江西	63.7	3.5	5.8	4.3	0.6	15.9
15	山东	166.7	1.0	0.6	12.8	0.6	5.4
16	河南	210.7	10.0	5.0	15.9	1.7	12.1
17	湖北	103.7	2.7	2.6	10.3	1.4	16.0
18	湖南	97.9	0.1	0.1	6.8	1.6	30.5
19	广东	198.0	1.3	0.7	15.8	0.5	3.5
20	广西	89.0	2.2	2.5	4.7	0.2	5.1
21	海南	16.2	0.7	4.2	1.1	0.1	8.7
22	重庆	51.9	0.2	0.4	2.9	0.2	7.6
23	四川	124.0	3.7	3.1	5.0	0.7	17.0
24	贵州	56.3	3.4	6.4	2.7	0.6	27.1
25	云南	72.5	7.4	11.4	3.6	0.9	31.6
26	西藏	0.2	−0.2	−48.1	0.0	0.0	—
27	陕西	76.6	1.0	1.4	4.3	0.9	27.5
28	甘肃	30.8	0.1	0.3	1.4	0.2	16.5
29	青海	8.1	0.0	0.3	2.7	2.4	812.9
30	宁夏	11.6	−0.3	−2.9	0.5	−0.1	−18.5
31	新疆	24.5	−0.1	−0.3	2.1	0.3	19.4
32	兵团	2.8	−0.2	−7.1	0.1	0.0	−12.6

附表 3　2018 年个人献血比例汇总表

序号	地区	/%	比 2017 年增长	
			/百分点	增长率 /%
1	北京	70.3	8.1	13.0
2	天津	85.1	-1.7	-1.9
3	河北	78.5	-1.7	-2.1
4	山西	80.3	-1.1	-1.3
5	内蒙古	85.2	3.4	4.2
6	辽宁	77.1	-0.7	-0.9
7	吉林	70.6	-0.7	-0.9
8	黑龙江	83.1	0.3	0.4
9	上海	35.5	-1.5	-4.1
10	江苏	64.1	1.3	2.1
11	浙江	51.8	3.4	7.0
12	安徽	78.7	-1.0	-1.2
13	福建	60.5	3.3	5.7
14	江西	65.9	-1.8	-2.6
15	山东	80.6	-2.7	-3.2
16	河南	83.1	-3.0	-3.5
17	湖北	87.6	-0.9	-1.0
18	湖南	71.7	4.4	6.5
19	广东	59.1	6.1	11.6
20	广西	74.6	2.5	3.5
21	海南	63.5	2.8	4.6
22	重庆	84.4	6.1	7.8
23	四川	62.8	-1.7	-2.7
24	贵州	83.5	7.1	9.3
25	云南	64.7	-1.1	-1.7
26	西藏	44.4	19.0	74.7
27	陕西	84.4	-3.8	-4.4
28	甘肃	70.6	-4.4	-5.9
29	青海	83.9	1.7	2.0
30	宁夏	83.8	-13.7	-14.1
31	新疆	84.4	-0.4	-0.4
32	兵团	99.2	4.8	5.0

附表 4　2018 年 400ml 献血占比情况汇总表

序号	地区	/%	比 2017 年增长	
			/ 百分点	增长率 /%
1	北京	67.8	−5.0	−6.9
2	天津	79.0	−1.8	−2.3
3	河北	81.0	−1.7	−2.1
4	山西	90.0	−0.4	−0.4
5	内蒙古	67.1	−0.9	−1.3
6	辽宁	74.9	−0.4	−0.5
7	吉林	55.5	2.1	3.9
8	黑龙江	80.9	0.3	0.4
9	上海	36.8	−1.2	−3.3
10	江苏	38.6	2.0	5.5
11	浙江	37.9	0.9	2.4
12	安徽	50.7	−1.8	−3.4
13	福建	49.0	1.7	3.7
14	江西	57.8	0.1	0.2
15	山东	63.0	−3.9	−5.8
16	河南	92.6	−0.5	−0.6
17	湖北	49.8	0.5	0.9
18	湖南	54.0	−0.1	−0.2
19	广东	45.1	0.4	0.9
20	广西	59.4	−0.2	−0.3
21	海南	52.3	1.4	2.8
22	重庆	54.5	−1.4	−2.4
23	四川	50.5	−1.6	−3.1
24	贵州	56.3	1.7	3.1
25	云南	34.7	9.0	34.9
26	西藏	5.2	1.0	24.0
27	陕西	67.3	−2.4	−3.4
28	甘肃	33.3	0.4	1.3
29	青海	81.0	3.7	4.7
30	宁夏	83.0	−2.3	−2.7
31	新疆	54.9	0.2	0.4
32	兵团	37.7	−2.2	−5.6

附表 5　2018 年女性献血者比例汇总表

序号	地区	/%	比 2017 年增长	
			/百分点	增长率 /%
1	北京	30.7	2.4	8.4
2	天津	25.6	0.6	2.5
3	河北	33.4	0.8	2.3
4	山西	30.2	−0.1	−0.2
5	内蒙古	34.7	−0.5	−1.3
6	辽宁	39.6	0.4	1.0
7	吉林	36.7	0.7	1.8
8	黑龙江	40.5	−0.3	−0.7
9	上海	30.4	0.3	1.2
10	江苏	39.4	0.6	1.5
11	浙江	38.3	0.5	1.2
12	安徽	40.4	0.3	0.7
13	福建	37.8	0.9	2.5
14	江西	39.0	0.7	1.7
15	山东	29.6	0.8	2.9
16	河南	37.0	−0.2	−0.4
17	湖北	38.1	0.8	2.1
18	湖南	39.6	1.8	4.9
19	广东	31.6	0.9	2.8
20	广西	34.9	1.0	2.9
21	海南	30.8	1.0	3.2
22	重庆	50.6	0.8	1.6
23	四川	48.1	1.2	2.5
24	贵州	51.4	2.0	4.1
25	云南	44.7	2.4	5.8
26	西藏	25.7	0.2	0.9
27	陕西	37.7	1.2	3.3
28	甘肃	31.1	1.0	3.2
29	青海	33.8	0.8	2.3
30	宁夏	36.5	0.5	1.4
31	新疆	33.9	1.5	4.7
32	兵团	34.7	1.9	5.7

附表 6 2018 年 18~35 岁献血者占比情况汇总表

序号	地区	/%	比 2017 年增长	
			/百分点	增长率 /%
1	北京	64.9	−2.0	−3.1
2	天津	70.5	0.1	0.2
3	河北	46.1	−1.1	−2.3
4	山西	42.9	−0.8	−1.7
5	内蒙古	45.8	−1.0	−2.1
6	辽宁	48.0	−0.2	−0.3
7	吉林	50.3	0.3	0.6
8	黑龙江	40.9	−0.7	−1.7
9	上海	73.3	0.0	0.0
10	江苏	50.9	−1.1	−2.2
11	浙江	53.7	−0.6	−1.2
12	安徽	52.0	−0.2	−0.5
13	福建	52.2	−1.1	−2.0
14	江西	56.1	0.5	0.9
15	山东	52.6	0.1	0.3
16	河南	40.1	−0.2	−0.6
17	湖北	52.9	−0.4	−0.7
18	湖南	54.5	0.0	0.1
19	广东	63.6	0.2	0.4
20	广西	53.7	0.2	0.4
21	海南	63.0	−0.2	−0.3
22	重庆	49.6	−1.2	−2.4
23	四川	43.0	−1.6	−3.6
24	贵州	56.2	0.1	0.2
25	云南	60.6	1.7	2.9
26	西藏	68.8	−5.3	−7.1
27	陕西	54.0	0.2	0.3
28	甘肃	58.1	−0.8	−1.4
29	青海	46.0	1.0	2.2
30	宁夏	55.3	−1.3	−2.3
31	新疆	57.4	2.3	4.2
32	兵团	57.0	0.2	0.4

附表 7　2018 年本科以上学历献血者占比情况汇总表

序号	地区	/%	比 2017 年增长	
			/ 百分点	增长率 /%
1	北京	34.6	7.9	29.4
2	天津	23.0	2.8	13.7
3	河北	15.3	1.1	7.4
4	山西	19.1	−0.5	−2.5
5	内蒙古	23.2	1.6	7.6
6	辽宁	21.0	0.3	1.6
7	吉林	24.2	1.6	7.2
8	黑龙江	21.3	−0.3	−1.2
9	上海	23.4	2.2	10.3
10	江苏	21.5	0.3	1.3
11	浙江	22.2	−0.3	−1.5
12	安徽	24.6	1.1	4.8
13	福建	29.1	1.1	3.8
14	江西	25.5	1.3	5.4
15	山东	19.8	1.2	6.6
16	河南	13.7	1.5	12.1
17	湖北	27.1	1.1	4.3
18	湖南	28.8	0.6	2.2
19	广东	19.3	1.2	6.4
20	广西	18.3	−0.2	−0.9
21	海南	28.8	0.7	2.3
22	重庆	21.0	0.7	3.7
23	四川	17.2	0.2	0.9
24	贵州	15.9	−1.6	−9.2
25	云南	24.3	2.5	11.5
26	西藏	21.4	−2.3	−9.7
27	陕西	21.7	1.4	6.7
28	甘肃	19.5	0.7	3.5
29	青海	19.6	1.0	5.5
30	宁夏	20.0	2.4	13.6
31	新疆	19.8	0.5	2.4
32	兵团	26.4	2.4	10.2

附表 8　2018 年血站血液检测情况汇总表

序号	地区	检测总数			不合格数			不合格率	
		/万人次	比 2017 年增长		/万人次	比 2017 年增长		/%	比 2017 年增长 /百分点
			/万人次	增长率 /%		/万人次	增长率 /%		
1	北京	41.2	−3.0	−6.9	6.1	−0.5	−7.3	14.8	−0.1
2	天津	21.8	1.0	4.9	2.8	−0.1	−4.0	12.6	−1.2
3	河北	89.8	3.5	4.0	10.4	0.0	0.3	11.5	−0.4
4	山西	42.0	2.0	5.0	6.2	−0.4	−6.2	14.7	−1.8
5	内蒙古	22.3	0.4	1.7	2.4	−0.3	−12.3	10.8	−1.7
6	辽宁	58.7	8.5	17.0	8.0	−0.3	−3.9	13.6	−2.9
7	吉林	29.8	0.7	2.4	3.1	−0.2	−5.9	10.6	−0.9
8	黑龙江	41.4	1.0	2.4	4.4	0.0	0.4	10.5	−0.2
9	上海	27.9	−0.4	−1.4	4.1	−0.2	−5.5	14.8	−0.7
10	江苏	111.7	4.9	4.6	9.5	0.3	3.1	8.5	−0.1
11	浙江	81.1	−0.4	−0.5	10.7	0.2	1.9	13.1	0.3
12	安徽	52.6	2.4	4.7	4.3	−0.2	−4.8	8.1	−0.8
13	福建	38.6	0.1	0.3	5.6	−0.3	−4.3	14.6	−0.7
14	江西	42.9	2.3	5.7	3.8	−0.4	−9.8	8.9	−1.5
15	山东	111.0	3.7	3.4	9.7	0.4	3.9	8.7	0.0
16	河南	127.7	5.7	4.7	12.6	0.2	1.4	9.9	−0.3
17	湖北	69.9	3.8	5.8	4.1	0.4	10.2	5.9	0.2
18	湖南	61.9	1.3	2.1	4.3	−0.2	−4.8	6.9	−0.5
19	广东	147.2	5.2	3.7	18.2	1.2	6.8	12.4	0.4
20	广西	61.1	3.6	6.2	6.2	0.0	0.2	10.2	−0.6
21	海南	12.1	0.5	4.3	1.9	0.2	13.5	15.4	1.2
22	重庆	38.8	0.8	2.2	5.6	−0.2	−3.0	14.4	−0.8
23	四川	85.2	2.4	2.9	10.5	0.1	0.6	12.3	−0.3
24	贵州	39.5	2.7	7.3	3.8	0.4	11.4	9.7	0.4
25	云南	54.8	5.1	10.4	7.1	1.5	26.5	12.9	1.6
26	西藏	0.3	−0.2	−42.6	0.1	−0.1	−27.3	50.1	10.5
27	陕西	51.0	1.2	2.4	4.3	−0.6	−11.5	8.5	−1.3
28	甘肃	22.5	−0.2	−0.7	2.3	−0.6	−20.4	10.1	−2.5

续表

序号	地区	检测总数			不合格数			不合格率	
		/万人次	比 2017 年增长		/万人次	比 2017 年增长		/%	比 2017 年增长 /百分点
			/万人次	增长率 /%		/万人次	增长率 /%		
29	青海	5.7	0.2	4.4	1.2	0.3	28.4	21.6	4.0
30	宁夏	7.3	0.1	1.8	1.1	0.0	2.0	15.5	0.0
31	新疆	17.6	−0.1	−0.5	2.2	0.0	−0.2	12.6	0.0
32	兵团	2.0	−0.1	−4.2	0.3	0.0	−16.1	12.8	−1.8

附表 9 2018 年献血前检测结果汇总表

序号	地区	检测总数			不合格数			不合格率	
		/万人次	比 2017 年增长		/万人次	比 2017 年增长		/%	比 2017 年增长 /百分点
			/万人次	增长率 /%		/万人次	增长率 /%		
1	北京	41.2	−3.0	−6.9	5.4	−0.4	−6.5	13.1	0.0
2	天津	21.8	1.0	4.9	2.5	−0.1	−2.3	11.6	−0.9
3	河北	89.8	3.5	4.0	9.3	0.3	2.9	10.4	−0.1
4	山西	42.0	2.0	5.0	5.3	−0.4	−6.8	12.7	−1.6
5	内蒙古	22.3	0.4	1.7	1.9	−0.3	−13.2	8.5	−1.5
6	辽宁	58.7	8.5	17.0	7.3	−0.2	−2.9	12.5	−2.6
7	吉林	29.8	0.7	2.4	2.7	−0.2	−5.3	9.2	−0.8
8	黑龙江	41.4	1.0	2.4	3.8	0.1	1.8	9.1	0.0
9	上海	27.9	−0.4	−1.4	2.8	0.0	0.0	10.0	0.1
10	江苏	111.7	4.9	4.6	8.1	0.4	5.8	7.3	0.1
11	浙江	81.1	−0.4	−0.5	9.7	0.3	2.8	11.9	0.4
12	安徽	52.6	2.4	4.7	3.2	0.0	0.3	6.2	−0.3
13	福建	38.6	0.1	0.3	4.9	−0.1	−1.6	12.6	−0.2
14	江西	42.9	2.3	5.7	3.0	−0.4	−11.2	7.1	−1.4
15	山东	111.0	3.7	3.4	7.9	0.5	6.4	7.1	0.2
16	河南	127.7	5.7	4.7	10.8	0.1	1.3	8.4	−0.3
17	湖北	69.9	3.8	5.8	2.7	0.5	25.3	3.9	0.6
18	湖南	61.9	1.3	2.1	2.9	0.0	−1.0	4.7	−0.1

序号	地区	检测总数			不合格数			不合格率	
		/万人次	比2017年增长		/万人次	比2017年增长		/%	比2017年增长/百分点
			/万人次	增长率/%		/万人次	增长率/%		
19	广东	147.2	5.2	3.7	14.0	1.4	10.9	9.5	0.6
20	广西	61.1	3.6	6.2	4.9	0.2	4.2	8.1	−0.2
21	海南	12.1	0.5	4.3	1.6	0.2	14.6	13.0	1.2
22	重庆	38.8	0.8	2.2	4.7	0.1	1.7	12.0	−0.1
23	四川	85.2	2.4	2.9	7.7	0.4	5.2	9.0	0.2
24	贵州	39.5	2.7	7.3	2.7	0.6	28.8	6.9	1.2
25	云南	54.8	5.1	10.4	5.9	1.6	36.6	10.8	2.1
26	西藏	0.3	−0.2	−42.6	0.1	0.0	−25.8	47.8	10.8
27	陕西	51.0	1.2	2.4	3.5	−0.4	−11.0	6.8	−1.0
28	甘肃	22.5	−0.2	−0.7	1.9	−0.5	−22.0	8.3	−2.3
29	青海	5.7	0.2	4.4	1.1	0.3	36.1	19.6	4.6
30	宁夏	7.3	0.1	1.8	1.1	0.0	4.6	14.5	0.4
31	新疆	17.6	−0.1	−0.5	1.8	0.0	1.1	10.5	0.2
32	兵团	2.0	−0.1	−4.2	0.2	0.0	−18.2	9.9	−1.7

附表10　2018年血液实验室检测情况汇总表

序号	地区	检测总数			不合格数			不合格率	
		/万份	比2017年增长		/万份	比2017年增长		/%	比2017年增长/百分点
			/万份	增长率/%		/万份	增长率/%		
1	北京	36.5	−2.0	−5.1	0.7	−0.1	−13.1	1.9	−0.2
2	天津	18.9	1.0	5.3	0.2	−0.1	−19.3	1.2	−0.4
3	河北	80.0	3.6	4.6	1.0	−0.2	−18.1	1.3	−0.4
4	山西	37.7	2.5	7.0	0.9	0.0	−2.4	2.3	−0.2
5	内蒙古	22.9	1.0	4.7	0.5	0.0	−9.0	2.2	−0.3
6	辽宁	42.7	−1.2	−2.6	0.6	−0.1	−13.9	1.5	−0.2

续表

序号	地区	检测总数			不合格数			不合格率	
		/万份	比 2017 年增长		/万份	比 2017 年增长		/%	比 2017 年增长 /百分点
			/万份	增长率 /%		/万份	增长率 /%		
7	吉林	26.9	0.8	3.2	0.4	0.0	−9.7	1.5	−0.2
8	黑龙江	37.9	1.2	3.3	0.6	0.0	−7.6	1.5	−0.2
9	上海	34.8	−0.3	−0.7	1.3	−0.2	−15.5	3.8	−0.7
10	江苏	104.7	4.8	4.8	1.3	−0.2	−11.0	1.3	−0.2
11	浙江	71.0	4.7	7.1	1.0	−0.1	−6.1	1.4	−0.2
12	安徽	49.7	0.8	1.7	1.0	−0.2	−17.7	2.1	−0.5
13	福建	34.3	0.2	0.7	0.8	−0.2	−18.1	2.3	−0.5
14	江西	39.5	2.3	6.2	0.8	0.0	−4.0	1.9	−0.2
15	山东	103.9	1.2	1.2	1.8	−0.1	−5.9	1.7	−0.1
16	河南	121.1	6.5	5.7	1.9	0.0	1.8	1.6	−0.1
17	湖北	71.9	2.2	3.2	1.4	−0.2	−10.2	2.0	−0.3
18	湖南	59.6	1.2	2.0	1.4	−0.2	−12.0	2.3	−0.4
19	广东	141.0	6.2	4.6	4.2	−0.2	−5.2	2.9	−0.3
20	广西	60.1	0.0	0.0	1.3	−0.2	−12.6	2.2	−0.3
21	海南	10.5	0.3	3.1	0.3	0.0	7.6	2.8	0.1
22	重庆	34.2	0.6	1.8	0.9	−0.3	−21.5	2.7	−0.8
23	四川	76.8	2.8	3.8	2.9	−0.3	−10.1	3.7	−0.6
24	贵州	39.8	1.6	4.1	1.1	−0.2	−16.4	2.8	−0.7
25	云南	48.6	3.7	8.3	1.1	−0.1	−8.8	2.3	−0.4
26	西藏	0.1	−0.2	−54.6	0.0	0.0	−48.5	4.5	0.5
27	陕西	47.5	1.7	3.6	0.9	−0.1	−13.4	1.8	−0.4
28	甘肃	21.3	−0.2	−0.8	0.4	−0.1	−11.9	1.9	−0.2
29	青海	4.8	0.0	−0.5	0.1	0.0	−17.5	2.4	−0.5
30	宁夏	6.5	−0.2	−3.3	0.1	0.0	−27.4	1.0	−0.3
31	新疆	17.9	−1.9	−9.4	0.4	0.0	−6.2	2.1	0.1
32	兵团	1.8	0.0	−2.0	0.1	0.0	−7.8	3.3	−0.2

附表 11 2018 年血液成分分离比例情况汇总表

序号	地区	/%	比 2017 年增长	
			/百分点	增长率 /%
1	北京	100.00	0.00	0.00
2	天津	99.82	0.01	0.01
3	河北	99.69	0.10	0.10
4	山西	99.71	0.07	0.07
5	内蒙古	99.32	−0.01	−0.01
6	辽宁	99.87	0.03	0.03
7	吉林	99.87	0.06	0.06
8	黑龙江	99.02	−0.31	−0.31
9	上海	99.86	0.07	0.07
10	江苏	99.97	0.02	0.02
11	浙江	99.88	0.02	0.02
12	安徽	99.86	0.08	0.08
13	福建	99.97	0.02	0.02
14	江西	100.00	0.01	0.01
15	山东	99.90	0.02	0.02
16	河南	99.82	−0.08	−0.08
17	湖北	99.94	0.01	0.01
18	湖南	100.00	0.01	0.01
19	广东	99.98	0.02	0.02
20	广西	99.99	0.00	0.00
21	海南	100.00	0.00	0.00
22	重庆	99.67	−0.23	−0.23
23	四川	99.98	0.07	0.07
24	贵州	99.94	−0.03	−0.03
25	云南	100.00	0.00	0.00
26	西藏	97.86	10.45	11.95
27	陕西	99.92	0.02	0.02
28	甘肃	99.77	0.03	0.03
29	青海	99.60	−0.07	−0.07
30	宁夏	97.22	−2.73	−2.73
31	新疆	96.80	−3.16	−3.16
32	兵团	97.69	−2.11	−2.11

附表 12   2018 年浓缩血小板分离率汇总表

序号	地区	/%	比 2017 年增长	
			/百分点	增长率 /%
1	北京	6.2	3.8	153.1
2	天津	10.6	3.6	50.4
3	河北	0.2	0.2	64 224.7
4	山西	0.8	0.0	4.0
5	内蒙古	8.4	3.3	64.6
6	辽宁	0.0	−0.1	−100.0
7	吉林	0.9	−1.9	−68.7
8	黑龙江	0.2	0.1	161.1
9	上海	0.9	−0.1	−5.3
10	江苏	0.2	0.1	36.1
11	浙江	0.2	0.2	1 121.8
12	安徽	5.0	0.4	8.7
13	福建	1.0	1.0	—
14	江西	0.6	0.2	46.2
15	山东	0.0	0.0	—
16	河南	0.2	0.0	−7.0
17	湖北	0.1	0.1	—
18	湖南	9.1	1.0	11.9
19	广东	7.7	3.8	97.2
20	广西	2.6	0.1	4.8
21	海南	0.0	0.0	—
22	重庆	0.0	0.0	28.5
23	四川	7.1	0.4	5.9
24	贵州	1.0	−0.8	−44.4
25	云南	0.0	0.0	−75.3
26	西藏	0.0	0.0	—
27	陕西	1.3	−0.4	−22.9
28	甘肃	0.0	0.0	−6.2
29	青海	6.4	1.5	29.2
30	宁夏	0.8	−2.4	−75.8
31	新疆	0.5	0.1	36.5
32	兵团	0.1	−0.5	−87.9

附表 13　2018 年供血总量汇总表

序号	地区	/万 U	比 2017 年增长	
			/万 U	增长率 /%
1	北京	128.1	2.3	1.8
2	天津	66.2	4.4	7.2
3	河北	251.1	7.7	3.2
4	山西	106.2	7.2	7.3
5	内蒙古	65.7	6.9	11.8
6	辽宁	127.2	−3.5	−2.7
7	吉林	78.8	2.4	3.2
8	黑龙江	122.7	12.2	11.0
9	上海	90.0	1.3	1.5
10	江苏	312.5	20.9	7.2
11	浙江	223.1	13.1	6.2
12	安徽	142.1	0.3	0.2
13	福建	97.1	0.4	0.4
14	江西	124.9	7.0	6.0
15	山东	311.8	1.0	0.3
16	河南	407.3	19.1	4.9
17	湖北	194.7	6.7	3.6
18	湖南	207.1	0.4	0.2
19	广东	445.9	90.3	25.4
20	广西	165.0	0.8	0.5
21	海南	27.9	0.9	3.3
22	重庆	99.8	9.2	10.2
23	四川	208.6	−1.9	−0.9
24	贵州	102.2	9.7	10.5
25	云南	135.7	18.0	15.3
26	西藏	1.0	0.2	33.1
27	陕西	146.2	1.9	1.3
28	甘肃	137.6	80.1	139.3
29	青海	18.6	0.0	0.0
30	宁夏	22.4	−1.0	−4.3
31	新疆	51.8	6.0	13.2
32	兵团	8.4	2.6	45.7

附表 14　2018 年万人血小板使用量汇总表

序号	地区	/治疗量	比 2017 年增长	
			/治疗量	增长率 /%
1	北京	52.21	3.25	6.6
2	天津	37.14	3.49	10.4
3	河北	14.27	1.03	7.8
4	山西	8.95	1.18	15.2
5	内蒙古	10.58	2.61	32.7
6	辽宁	12.02	−0.25	−2.0
7	吉林	10.22	0.58	6.0
8	黑龙江	9.72	0.50	5.4
9	上海	19.65	1.03	5.5
10	江苏	19.57	1.66	9.3
11	浙江	17.24	1.81	11.7
12	安徽	6.48	0.71	12.2
13	福建	9.52	0.67	7.5
14	江西	9.11	1.02	12.6
15	山东	12.73	0.70	5.8
16	河南	16.61	1.78	12.0
17	湖北	17.13	2.32	15.6
18	湖南	10.98	2.43	28.4
19	广东	15.17	1.24	8.9
20	广西	9.97	0.56	5.9
21	海南	12.01	1.03	9.3
22	重庆	9.06	0.76	9.1
23	四川	6.95	0.97	16.3
24	贵州	7.87	1.58	25.2
25	云南	7.43	1.85	33.3
26	西藏	0.00	0.00	—
27	陕西	11.34	2.40	26.9
28	甘肃	5.08	0.93	22.5
29	青海	44.64	−3.72	−7.7
30	宁夏	7.76	−1.51	−16.2
31	新疆	7.30	0.20	2.7
32	兵团	2.98	−0.35	−10.5

附表 15　2018 年有形成分利用率汇总表

序号	地区	/%	比 2017 年增长	
			/百分点	增长率 /%
1	北京	106.2	3.8	3.7
2	天津	110.4	3.6	7.8
3	河北	99.8	0.2	0.5
4	山西	100.5	0.1	0.2
5	内蒙古	107.7	3.3	5.4
6	辽宁	99.9	0.0	−0.1
7	吉林	100.7	−1.9	−3.5
8	黑龙江	99.2	−0.2	−0.3
9	上海	100.8	0.0	0.0
10	江苏	100.2	0.1	0.1
11	浙江	100.1	0.2	0.5
12	安徽	104.9	0.5	0.9
13	福建	101.0	1.0	1.9
14	江西	100.6	0.2	0.4
15	山东	99.9	0.0	0.1
16	河南	100.0	−0.1	−0.2
17	湖北	100.0	0.1	0.1
18	湖南	109.1	1.0	2.0
19	广东	107.6	3.8	7.0
20	广西	102.6	0.1	0.2
21	海南	100.0	0.0	0.0
22	重庆	99.7	−0.2	−0.4
23	四川	107.1	0.5	0.8
24	贵州	100.9	−0.8	−1.4
25	云南	100.0	0.0	−0.1
26	西藏	97.9	10.4	15.6
27	陕西	101.2	−0.4	−0.7
28	甘肃	99.8	0.0	0.1
29	青海	106.0	1.4	3.1
30	宁夏	98.0	−5.1	−9.8
31	新疆	97.3	−3.0	−5.8
32	兵团	97.8	−2.6	−5.2

附表 16 2018 年血液物理报废汇总表

序号	地区	物理报废量			报废率	
		/千 U	比 2017 年增长		/%	比 2017 年增长
			/千 U	增长率 /%		/ 百分点
1	北京	3.3	0.3	10.2	0.3	0.0
2	天津	2.7	0.7	38.4	0.4	0.1
3	河北	90.1	10.2	12.8	3.4	0.3
4	山西	106.3	16.1	17.9	8.9	0.7
5	内蒙古	54.0	−1.5	−2.7	7.5	−1.0
6	辽宁	76.2	−3.0	−3.8	5.6	−0.1
7	吉林	5.8	1.5	33.5	0.7	0.2
8	黑龙江	5.2	−0.7	−11.8	0.4	−0.1
9	上海	16.7	1.1	7.3	1.8	0.1
10	江苏	4.0	−0.6	−12.5	0.1	0.0
11	浙江	39.3	3.1	8.6	1.7	0.0
12	安徽	113.1	17.2	17.9	7.2	1.0
13	福建	57.4	−8.2	−12.5	5.4	−0.7
14	江西	43.6	8.2	23.1	3.3	0.5
15	山东	5.7	−0.7	−11.1	0.2	0.0
16	河南	58.9	1.4	2.4	1.4	0.0
17	湖北	88.9	7.8	9.6	4.3	0.2
18	湖南	50.7	−10.0	−16.5	2.3	−0.5
19	广东	233.9	−51.7	−18.1	4.9	−2.3
20	广西	69.9	12.1	21.0	4.0	0.7
21	海南	0.2	0.0	17.7	0.1	0.0
22	重庆	22.6	2.4	12.0	2.2	0.0
23	四川	171.8	−14.1	−7.6	7.3	−0.5
24	贵州	49.5	−15.1	−23.4	4.5	−1.8
25	云南	77.5	7.3	10.4	5.3	−0.2
26	西藏	0.2	0.0	3.3	2.0	−0.5

续表

序号	地区	物理报废量			报废率	
		/千U	比 2017 年增长		/%	比 2017 年增长
			/千U	增长率/%		/百分点
27	陕西	6.6	−3.5	−34.5	0.4	−0.2
28	甘肃	20.5	−3.4	−14.4	1.5	−2.5
29	青海	1.2	0.3	36.1	0.6	0.2
30	宁夏	4.4	1.3	40.7	1.9	0.6
31	新疆	29.8	3.0	11.3	5.3	−0.1
32	兵团	2.1	0.1	2.5	2.4	−0.9

附表 17　2018 年各主要城市血液采集情况

地市级行政区划	千人口献血率 / 千人口 $^{-1}$	人均采血量 /ml	人均采血小板量 / U·万人口 $^{-1}$
北京市	16.4	5.5	40.9
天津市	12.2	4.4	35.4
石家庄市	17.7	6.5	30.8
太原市	24.1	9.1	36.5
呼和浩特市	10.1	3.4	18.5
沈阳市	14.1	5.2	24.9
长春市	14.9	5.0	23.7
哈尔滨市	14.4	5.3	21.0
上海市	14.8	4.1	18.6
南京市	22.7	7.3	51.6
杭州市	18.2	5.6	40.9
合肥市	14.7	4.5	17.7
福州市	11.2	3.9	19.6
南昌市	20.3	6.8	26.3
济南市	18.4	6.1	32.1
郑州市	23.4	8.4	63.3

续表

地市级行政区划	千人口献血率 / 千人口 $^{-1}$	人均采血量 /ml	人均采血小板量 / U·万人口 $^{-1}$
武汉市	20.3	6.6	64.3
长沙市	19.5	7.0	31.1
广州市	25.3	8.1	46.7
南宁市	18.6	6.1	27.4
海口市	27.1	8.7	45.2
重庆市	11.0	3.5	8.7
成都市	13.9	4.8	23.1
贵阳市	21.0	6.5	29.0
昆明市	25.0	8.3	38.8
拉萨市	2.7	0.6	—
西安市	18.3	6.4	30.2
兰州市	16.1	4.9	27.7
西宁市	15.6	7.8	112.1
银川市	18.4	6.9	20.9
乌鲁木齐市	15.5	4.7	37.4
深圳市	12.9	4.5	22.2
大连市	12.2	3.9	17.5
青岛市	12.7	4.4	20.4
宁波市	11.5	3.4	14.7
厦门市	13.8	4.0	19.4

China's
Report on
Blood Safety
2018

National Health Commission of the People's Republic of China

Introduction

2018 marked the 20th anniversary of the promulgation and implementation of the *Law of Blood Donation of the People's Republic of China*. Over the past 20 years, the legal system of voluntary non-remunerated blood donation has been continuously improved, as has the blood service system. In addition, the blood supply and its safety has been effectively guaranteed. In 2018, China focused on improving law-based governance, enhancing blood supply, boosting the level of blood safety and increasing the rational use of blood, building a blood safety system that is reliable, equitable, accessible and characterized by quality-assurance and rational use.

I. Continuous Improvement of the Law-Based Governance of Blood Safety

As of 2018, all provinces (as well as autonomous regions and municipalities directly under the central government) formulated regulations or measures for the implementation of the *Law of Blood Donation*. 13 provincial capital cities and 14 cities with independent legislative jurisdiction have promulgated regulations or measures for blood donation at the municipal level. A legal system of voluntary non-remunerated blood donation at the national, provincial and municipal levels has been preliminarily established to ensure that there are laws and rules to follow when managing blood safety. The design framework of the blood safety technical standard system was completed in 2018. Four industry standards were issued at the same time. Important progress was

Note: Laws, regulations, notices, opinions, measures, reles, guidelines and standards published by the Chinese central and local authorities are in italics in this report.

also made in the blood technical standard system.

II. Innovative Incentive Mechanisms for Voluntary Non-remunerated Blood Donation

Innovative incentive mechanisms for voluntary non-remunerated blood donation have been explored all over the country. Models for the publicity and recruitment of volunteer blood donors have been expanded. The National Health Commission of China, the Red Cross Society of China and the Health Bureau of the Logistics and Support Department of the Central Military Commission appointed four national ambassadors for voluntary non-remunerated blood donation for the first time, to promote the humanitarian spirit to heal the wounded and save the dying through voluntary non-remunerated blood donation. On the 20th anniversary of the implementation of the *Law of Blood Donation*, 304 high-performing blood collection teams from the country were commended. All provinces (as well as autonomous regions and municipalities directly under the central government) coordinated closely and innovated new publicity and education models for voluntary blood donation in line with local characteristics. Effective measures were rolled out to guarantee the rights and interests of blood donors, facilitating fee reductions and exemptions for clinical and non-local blood transfusion expenses incurred by voluntary non-remunerated donors, and contributing to a positive social atmosphere of voluntary non-remunerated blood donation.

III. Optimization of the Blood Collection and Supply Service System

In 2018, basic factors such as the usable and constructed floor space for blood services were expanded in the country, achieving a total area of about 2.16 million square meters, an increase of 2.7% over 2017. The number of blood donation rooms and vehicles and other service facilities continued to rise, reaching 1,458 donation rooms, up by 5.65% over 2017. With the upgrade of instruments and equipment for laboratory testing and blood preparation, as well as the restructuring of blood services personnel, the proportion of highly educated health technicians was increased. With the improvement of information infrastructure, 26 provinces achieved network connectivity between blood service and blood donation sites, establishing a blood quality management information system covering the whole process of blood collection and supply from blood vessel to blood vessel.

IV. Expansion of Blood Supply Capacity

In 2018, the total number of voluntary non-remunerated donors, the total amount of donated blood and the rate of donation per thousand people reached new highs, registering 14.79 million donations, 25.06 million donated units and a rate of 11.1 per 1,000, respectively. The separation rate of blood components was 99.82%. In addition, the supply of erythrocyte reached 22.67 million units, an increase of 2.8% over 2017. 1.779 million units of platelets and 21.322 million units of plasma components were collected, an increase of 10.2% and 12.4% over 2017, respectively. In 2018, the Blood Center of the Xizang Zizhiqu Autonomous Region initiated blood nucleic acid testing, ending the historical lack of a nucleic acid testing laboratory in Xizang Zizhiqu. These measures effectively guaranteed the blood safety in local areas.

(Remark: the data of this report do not include HONG KONG SAR, MACAU SAR and TAIWAN Province)

2018 年国家血液安全报告
China's Report on Blood Safety 2018

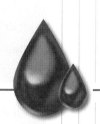

Legislative Development for Blood Safety

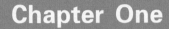

Chapter One

Legislative Development for Blood Management

I. Improvement of the Local Legislative Framework Has Offered Strong Legal Guarantee for Blood Safety.

The promulgation and implementation of the *Law of Blood Donation of the People's Republic of China* (hereinafter referred to as the "*Law of Blood Donation*") has provided the legal basis for blood management in China. The legislative bodies of various provinces, cities and local governments have been putting forward measures, rules and regulations to facilitate implementation of the *Law of Blood Donation*. A three-tier legal framework has gradually taken shape, with the *Law of Blood Donation* at the top, the provincial implementation regulations in the middle and the municipal and local measures at the bottom.

Since the promulgation and implementation of the *Law of Blood Donation* in 1998, 31 provinces (as well as autonomous regions and municipalities directly under the central government) in China had circulated regulations or measures for the implementation of the *Law of Blood Donation* by 2018. Among them, a total of 8 provinces (as well as autonomous regions and municipalities directly under the central government), including Beijing, Hebei, Shanghai, Zhejiang, Shandong, Guangdong, Guangxi and Hainan, completed the first revision of their local legislations. Jiangsu and Chongqing carried out their second revisions. In 2018, Hainan launched their first revision. Guangdong and Chongqing completed the revision in 2017 and started implementation in

2018., showing in Table 1-1.

Table 1-1   List of local legislations and revisions(Part)

No.	Region	Title of Measures or Regulations	Year of Promulgation	Revision Status	
				First Revision	Second Revision
1	Beijing	Measures of Beijing Municipality on the administration of blood donation and transfusion by citizens/Measures of Beijing Municipality on the administration of blood donation	1999	2009	—
2	Hebei	Measures of Hebei Province on the implementation of the blood donation law of the people's Republic of China	2000	2010	—
3	Shanghai	Regulations of Shanghai Municipality on blood donation	1998	2010	—
4	Jiangsu	Regulations of Jiangsu Province on blood donation	2000	2010	2017
5	Zhejiang	Measures of Zhejiang Province for the implementation of the blood donation law of the people's Republic of China	2001	2013	—
6	Shandong	Measures of Shandong Province for the implementation of the blood donation law of the people's Republic of China	2000	2004	—
7	Guangdong	Measures of Guangdong Province for the implementation of the blood donation law of the people's Republic of China	1998	2017	—
8	Guangxi	Regulations of Guangxi Zhuangzu Zizhiqu on blood donation	2001	2010	—
9	Hainan	Regulations of Hainan Special Economic Zone on blood donation without compensation	2012	2018 (launched)	—
10	Chongqing	Regulations of Chongqing Municipality on blood donation	1998	2010	2017

With the promotion of provincial-level legislations, the corresponding local measures for the implementation of the *Law of Blood Donation* were publicized in different places. As of 2018, 13 provincial capitals, including Ürümqi, Xi'an, Hangzhou and Jinan, promulgated measures to implement the *Law of Blood Donation* at the municipal level, among which the legislations of Xi'an, Shenyang and Nanning were revised for the first time, and the legislations of Kunming were revised for the second time (Table 1-2). It has effectively guaranteed the local implementation of the *Law of Blood Donation* to enhance blood safety. Local legislations at all levels contribute to the lawful governance for blood safety.

Table 1-2　Legislations by provincial capitals (ranking by the year of promulgation)

No.	City	Title of Measures or Regulations	Year of Promulgation	Year of Revision
1	Ürümqi	*Regulations of Ürümqi Municipality on voluntary blood donation*	1993	Repealed
2	Xi'an	*Measures of Guiyang Municipality on the administration of the use of blood by citizens*	1998	2013
3	Hangzhou	*Measures of Hangzhou Municipality on the implementation of the Law of Blood Donation of the People's Republic of China*	1999	—
4	Ji'nan	*Regulations of Jinan on the administration of blood donation*	2001	—
5	Shenyang	*Measures of Shenyang Municipality on the administration of blood donation*	2001	2016
6	Wuhan	*Regulations of Wuhan Municipality on blood donation*	2002	—
7	Kunming	*Measures of Kunming Municipality on the administration of blood donation* *Regulations of Kunming Municipality on blood donation*	2002	2008 2018
8	Guangzhou	*Regulations of Guangzhou Municipality on the administration of blood donation*	2004	—
9	Nanning	*Regulations of Nanning Municipality on blood donation*	2004	2012

Continued

No.	City	Title of Measures or Regulations	Year of Promulgation	Year of Revision
10	Chengdu	*Measures of Chengdu Municipality for the implementation of the blood donation law of the people's Republic of China*	2011	—
11	Guiyang	*Measures of Guiyang Municipality on the administration of the use of blood by citizens*	2011	—
12	Taiyuan	*Regulations of Taiyuan Municipality on blood donation*	2015	—
13	Nanjing	*Regulations of Nanjing Municipality on blood donation*	2017	—

Among the 22 cities with independent legislative jurisdiction in China, 14 have promulgated blood donation regulations or measures. Qingdao, Xiamen, Fushun, Suzhou, Xuzhou, Ningbo and Tangshan have revised their local legislations for the first time. Other cities, such as Zibo and Dalian, have repealed their outdated legislations (Table 1-3).

Table 1-3   Legislations by cities with independent legislative jurisdiction (ranking by the year of promulgation)

No.	City	Title of Measures or Regulations	Year of Promulgation	Year of Latest Revision
1	Qiqihar	*Regulations of Qiqihar Municipality on the administration of blood donation and transfusion by citizens*	1996	—
2	Qingdao	*Regulations of Qingdao Municipality on voluntary blood donation*	1996	2003
3	Zibo	*Measures of Zibo Municipality on the administration of voluntary non-remunerated blood donation by citizens*	1997	2010 (repealed)
4	Xiamen	*Regulations of Xiamen Special Economic Zone on unpaid blood donation*	1997	2009
5	Fushun	*Interim Measures of Fushun City for the implementation of the Law of Blood Donation of the People's Republic of China*	1998	2002

Continued

No.	City	Title of Measures or Regulations	Year of Promulgation	Year of Latest Revision
6	Suzhou	*Regulations of Suzhou Municipality on blood donation*	1999	2015
7	Wuxi	*Measures of Wuxi Municipality on the administration of blood donation*	1999	—
8	Xuzhou	*Regulations of Xuzhou Municipality on voluntary blood donation*	1999	2015
9	Ningbo	*Regulations of Ningbo Municipality on blood donation*	1999	2012
10	Dalian	*Regulations of Dalian Municipality on blood donation*	2000	2010 (repealed)
11	Tangshan	*Regulations of Tangshan Municipality on blood donation*	2004	2010
12	Datong	*Regulations of Datong City on blood donation*	2007	—
13	Jilin	*Regulations of Jilin Municipality on unpaid blood donation*	2014	—
14	Shenzhen	*Regulations of Shenzhen Special Economic Zone on unpaid blood donation*	2015	—

II. Innovation Was Made in the Scope of Local Legislation and Support for Blood Safety Was Improved.

In 2018, some provinces and cities carried out exploration and innovation from the top-level design and working mechanism in response to the challenges and problems in blood security. Local legislative efforts exhibited new momentum at all levels. **First, the responsibilities of relevant government departments were clarified.** The feasibility and effectiveness of lawful practice was enhanced. For example, the *Regulations of Hainan Special Economic Zone on voluntary non-remunerated blood donation* (hereinafter referred to as *the Hainan Regulations*) clearly defines the responsibilities of people's governments at all levels, departments of finance, departments of public security and urban management, departments of transportation, departments of education, human resources and social security and other relevant organs. The *Regulations* *of Kunming on blood donation* (hereinafter referred to as the *Kunming Regulations*) makes it clear that the leadership of the people's government of the city, county (as well as prefecture and district) on blood donation will be included in the annual performance evaluation objectives. The responsibilities of relevant departments were clarified. **Second, social awareness of voluntary non-remunerated blood donation was raised.** According to the *Hainan Regulations*, "January is the public campaign month for voluntary non-remunerated blood donation in this special economic zone every year". The *Kunming Regulations* stipulates that "January is the voluntary blood donation month for medical professionals, and February is for civil servants. Other months are allocated by the Municipal People's government." **Third, the rights and interests of blood donors were protected.** According to the *Hainan Regulations*, voluntary non-remunerated blood donors and their relatives have the right to priority service of blood transfusion. "On the premise of ensuring the clinical emergency in blood transfusion, medical institutions should give priority to donors, their spouses, parents and children for clinical use of blood". The eligible blood donors and volunteers can enjoy the "three exemptions". "Individuals who donate blood in the special economic zone and have won the national voluntary non-remunerated blood donation award, the national award for voluntary non-remunerated donation of blood stem cell and the national lifetime honor award for volunteer service in blood donation can enjoy the following preferential treatments in the special economic zone with relevant proof of certificates: (1) exemption of admission fees for visiting scenic spots invested and constructed by the state; (2) exemption of outpatient registration fees and medical examination fees at public medical institutions; (3) free ride on urban rail transit and buses; (4) entitlements to other preferential treatments stipulated by the provincial people's government". According to the *Kunming Regulations*, the eligible blood donors and volunteers can enjoy the treatment of "three preferential treatments, four exemptions and one subsidy". Specifically, it means "(1) preferential treatments in employment and referral, guarantee children's enrollment at kindergartens and elementary schools under the same conditions; (2) exemption from admission fees to government-sponsored parks, scenic spots and other amenities, from outpatient registration and examination fees at public medical institutions, priority diagnosing and treating; a free physical examination with the basic items provided by the blood-receiving medical institutions; and free rides on urban rail transit and buses; (3) a social security subsidy to those without stable income". **Fourth, breakthrough and innovation were achieved.** As the only provincial-level special economic zone in China, Hainan has greater flexibility and autonomy in legislation. In the process of amending the regulations, Hainan studied the characteristics of the region and achieved some breakthroughs and innovations. First, the age limit for eligible blood donors was lifted to 65 years old. "If a repeat blood donor has no previous negative reaction to donation and meets the requirements of health examination to donate again, the age limit can be extended to 65 years old". Second, the intervals between donations were adjusted. "The interval between two collections shall be no less than 3 months for men and 4 months for women". Third, the cost of autotransfusion was able to covered in the health insurance. "The cost of autotransfusion of blood users shall be included in the coverage scope of basic health insurance in accordance with relevant regulations". The revision of the regulations has greatly improved the sense of honor and tangible benefits for donors and volunteers. It not only makes donors feel the loving care of the society, but also plays an exemplary role in rousing the enthusiasm of healthy citizens of appropriate age to participate in voluntary non-remunerated blood donation.

Chapter Two

Formulating Industry Standards for Blood Transfusion

Since the establishment of the Blood Standards Sub-Committee of the National Health Standards Committee in 1996, standardization of blood transfusion in China has been making great strides. At present, there are 2 national standards and 10 industrial standards (Table 1-4).

Table1-4   Standards for blood transfusion

Category	Titles of Standards
National standards	*Requirements for health examination of blood donors (GB 18467—2011)*
	Quality requirements for whole blood and component blood (GB 18469—2012)
Industry standards	*Common terms of transfusion medicine (WS/T 203—2001)*
	Requirements for configuration of blood establishments (WS/T 401—2012)
	Blood storage requirements (WS 399—2012)
	Blood transport requirements (WS/T 400—2012)
	Guidelines for quality monitoring of whole blood and component blood (WS/T 550—2017)
	Guidelines for classification of adverse reactions in blood donation (WS/T 551—2017)
	Guidelines for prevention and treatment of vasovagal responses related to blood donation (WS/T 595—2018)
	Internal blood transfusion (WS/T 622—2018)
	Use of whole blood and component blood (WS/T 623—2018)
	Classification of blood transfusion reactions (WS/T 624—2018)

I. A Basic Framework for Blood Transfusion Standards

The establishment of a blood transfusion standard system is the basis of standardized management of collection and supply for clinical blood transfusion. It promotes the development of the blood transfusion industry and technical progress. According to the newly revised *Standardization Law of the People's Republic of China* in 2018, a new framework for blood transfusion standards was built on the basis of the original standard system. The new framework rebuilt the overall hierarchical structure of the standard system, including eight layers: the blood foundation, blood donation service, blood preparation, blood supply, blood detection, clinical blood transfusion, quality management and information system of the blood transfusion service. It improved the systematization, coordination and applicability of blood transfusion standards. Among the four trade standards released in 2018, *Guidelines for prevention and treatment of vasovagal responses related to blood donation* is related to blood donation service. *Use of whole blood and component blood, Internal blood transfusion and Classification of blood transfusion reactions* are related to clinical blood transfusion. At the same time, blood preparation and other standards are continuously advancing. The professional committee of blood standards managed the system framework dynamically, adjusted the system according to the latest development of the international standardization system in the blood industry, and promoted the structure and systematization of China's blood transfusion standards.

II. Improved Evidence-based Standards

With the great progress made in blood transfusion standardization in China, a standard-making pattern was formed, with "the government playing a leading role, active participation from the industry, and alignment with both national conditions and international benchmarks". The criteria for standard formulation were established, requiring that all views be evidence-based, all data clearly sourced. By referring to the relevant foreign standards and targeted, professional and scientific research, the formulation process was increasingly standard, evidence-based and reasonable. The *Guidelines for prevention and treatment of vasovagal responses related to blood donation* issued in 2018 has made clear requirements for the identification, prevention and treatment measures for donors prone to adverse reactions, and facilities needed at the blood establishment, which provides theoretical basis and technical guidance for the prevention and treatment of adverse reactions blood donation by the blood establishment staff. *"Use of whole blood and component blood"* is the first blood use standard in China. The expert group carried out research for more than 3 years and referred to a large number of relevant standards at home and abroad. It made new and more evidence-based and reasonable requirements and regulations on the indications, dosage and use methods of whole blood and component blood, and classification of blood transfusion reaction. It marked the start of standardized blood use in China. *Internal blood transfusion and Classification of blood transfusion reactions* are standards to guide clinical use of blood. The release of these 3 trade standards played an important role in promoting the treatment and evaluation of clinical transfusion and rational use of blood in clinical situations at medical institutions. It also provided basis for the supervision and evaluation of health administrative departments. The continuous update and improvement of blood transfusion standards would help regulate and guide better practice and promote the sustainable development of the industry.

2018 年国家血液安全报告
China's Report on Blood Safety 2018

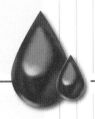

Social
Awareness of
Voluntary Non-
Remunerated
Blood Donation

In 2018, the National Health Commission issued *a notice on organizing and carrying out awareness campaigns of the World Blood Donor Day*, (National Health Commission Office Medical Notice [2018] No. 238) and *a notice on carrying out the summary and publicity activities of the 20th anniversary of the implementation of the Law of Blood Donation* (National Health Commission Office Medical Notice [2018] No. 483). The publicity and recruitment of voluntary non-remunerated blood donors were prompted all over the country, raising social awareness and support. The cause of voluntary non-remunerated blood donation became widely and warmly supported by the whole society. More and more citizens with compassion joined in the ranks of voluntary non-remunerated blood donors. The cause of voluntary non-remunerated blood donation cause showed a healthy, sustainable and encouraging momentum.

Chapter one

Publicity of Voluntary Non-remunerated Blood Donation

I. Publicity of Voluntary Non-remunerated Blood Donation Increased.

On June 14, 2018, the promotional poster of the 15th World Blood Donor Day was officially released by the National Health Commission of China, the Red Cross Society of China and the Health Bureau of the Logistics and Support Department of the Central Military Commission. Hai Xia, Wu Jing, Zhang Han, and Jian Renzi were presented as national ambassadors for voluntary non-remunerated blood donation. The National Health Commission of China, the Red Cross Society of China and the Health Bureau of the Logistics and Support Department of the Central Military Commission also jointly produced a public service film on voluntary non-remunerated blood donation. The publicity promoted the healthy and steady development of the great undertaking of voluntary non-remunerated blood donation to the benefit of public welfare. A series of official slogans were launched successively, including "Donate blood, the gift of life" "Be a donor. Be their hero", and "The moment you reach out your arm, you become the focus of the crowd". Entrusted by the National Health Commission, Wuhan province hosted the main celebration of the World Blood Donor Day in China.

With increasing public awareness and publicity of voluntary non-remunerated blood donation at the national level, various provinces also responded proactively. On the one hand, the selfless and heroic acts of voluntary non-remunerated blood donors were vigorously publicized through traditional media, such as newspaper, radio, television, poster and car advertisement . On the other hand, those voluntary non-remunerated blood donors were spread through digital and social media, such as Internet, WeChat, Weibo (microblog). More audience was reached through innovative models and expansive channels, building a comprehensive three-dimensional communication system in a way that is popular with the public. The research data on the promotion of voluntary non-remunerated blood donation in 27 provinces (as well as municipalities directly under the central government) showed that all blood establishments had open days. For instance, Hainan province holds open days more than once a month, helping public understanding and knowledge of blood donation. 26 provinces and cities carried out acknowledgement events for selfless individual donors. Ambassadors for voluntary non-remunerated blood donation were recommended in 19 provinces and cities. In Jiangxi province, a grand celebration was carried out to commend the Compassion of Blood Donors in Passing on the Love of the City and to Commemorate the 20th Anniversary of the Implementation of the *Law of Blood Donation*. Thirty ambassadors for voluntary non-remunerated blood donation communication were selected by way of a quiz on blood donation knowledge. The microfilms and promotional films about voluntary non-remunerated blood donation produced in many provinces attracted wide attention, especially that of the young people.

II. Brilliant Publicity Activities for Voluntary Non-remunerated Blood Donation Were Arranged.

2018 marked the 20th anniversary of the promulgation of the *Law of Blood Donation*. A host of activities around the 20th anniversary of the *Law of Blood Donation* was held in different provinces. Public awareness and publicity of voluntary non-remunerated blood donation were promoted, creating an encouraging social atmosphere. With the strong support from the Communist Party of China provincial committees and governments, improved publicity and recruitment forms were utilized in institutions, enterprises, schools, villages and communities. Among them, some leagues and cities in Nei Mongol Zizhiqu extended the publicity activities for voluntary non-remunerated blood donation all the way down to pastures and horse farms, and carried out voluntary non-remunerated blood donation volunteer-recruitment based on specific local conditions. Innovative models such as lectures, experience-sharing and knowledge contests on voluntary non-remunerated blood donation were adopted by some regions to strengthen the publicity and education of voluntary non-remunerated blood donation, as well as to promote the humanitarian spirit of medicine, i.e. healing the wounded and saving the dying. According to the research results of voluntary non-remunerated blood donation promotion in 26 provinces and cities, all of them had launched exclusive blood donation bus routes. 20 provinces and cities had carried out survey on the awareness of voluntary non-remunerated blood donation among urban residents and students. See Table 2-1 for the detailed publicity activities for the 20th anniversary celebration by each province.

Table 2-1   Provincial publicity activities for the 20th anniversary
of the Law of Blood Donation

Region	Activities
Heilongjiang	More than 150 publicity activities on campuses and in communities, organizations, enterprises and rural areas. Special reports on 27 provincial volunteers who won the national lifetime honor award for voluntary non-remunerated blood donation in the mainstream media. Publicity campaigns for voluntary non-remunerated blood donation were carried out on college and university campuses across the province, with the theme of "Twenty years of unity and solidarity by Chinese blood donors"
Qinghai	Around the theme of building a healthy province and deepening healthcare reform, various forms of publicity and reports were carried out, with 106 pieces of information communicated throughout the year "Blood doors are heroes" and other themed publicity activities
Fujian	Publicity and education activities with the theme of "Twenty years of unity and solidarity by Chinese blood donors"
Hunan	Revision of local blood donation measures
Hubei	Hosted the "Shining Red" national blood establishment speech event
Hainan	Incorporate the revision of the regulations of Hainan Special Economic Zone on free blood donation into the legislative plan "Run for blood and health" campaign

Continued

Region	Activities
Jiangsu	More than 2,500 events of "five promotions" at blood collection and supply institutions in the whole province Publicity month focusing on mutual love and bond for voluntary non-remunerated blood donation Publicity and recruitment activities such as speech competition series, "Listen to my story", at blood collection and supply institutions
The Xinjiang Production and Construction Crops	Themed activities of "Twenty years of unity and solidarity by Chinese blood donors" Training on blood donation laws, regulations and related knowledge
Guangdong	Themed activities of "donate blood and share life"
Shandong	Production of public service advertisement "Blood Fate" and micro film "Life Express"
Anhui	Celebrating the World Blood Donor Day and the 20th anniversary of the implementation of the Law of Blood Donation of the People's Republic of China Province-wide selection of blood donation stars, both individuals and organizations.
Tianjin	Large-scale non-profit run of "Blood from Tianjin, love for all"
Sichuan	Give full play to the celebrity effect, with voluntary non-remunerated blood donation as one of the themes of the second season of "Li Boqing's health talk shows" Winter publicity activity for voluntary non-remunerated blood donation for public servants in 2018 Walking activity with the theme of "healthy life and happy blood donation"
Yunnan	"Voluntary non-remunerated blood donation: boundless love-you are legend 2018" essay campaign "818, Helping Panda Man" Kunming rare blood donation campaign
Shanghai	Issued the *notice on carrying out a series of activities to commemorate the 20th anniversary of the implementation of the Law of Blood Donation of the People's Republic of China and "Regulations of Shanghai Municipality on blood donation"*; Hand-painted posters to commemorate the 20th anniversary of the law A special film by Shanghai Municipality on 20 years of voluntary non-remunerated blood donation Produced the 2018 story collection of excellent volunteers for voluntary non-remunerated blood donation Edited and produced a monthly special edition in the Xinmin Evening News, *Blood and Life*

In order to better publicize voluntary non-remunerated blood donation and foster a caring and loving social climate for voluntary non-remunerated blood donation, China Blood Transfusion Association, Hubei Provincial Speech Association and Wuhan Blood Center jointly launched the national blood centers reporting and presentation event named "Shining Red". 30 provincial and municipal blood centers participated in the event. With enormous enthusiasm and touching stories, the contestants showcased the positiveness and passion of all the blood center workers. Overwhelmed the audience with their interpretation of the selfless blood donation, the reporting and presentation were to attract and call on more groups and individuals with a sense of social responsibility to participate in the vigorous development of voluntary non-remunerated blood donation.

III. Voluntary Non-remunerated Blood Donation Had Received Growing Attention

In 2018, voluntary non-remunerated blood donation publicity activities at all levels in China had received increasing attention, which resulted in a positive social impact. The public put the awareness of blood donation in the new era into real actions in a loving and selfless manner, during which many amazing stories had happened. On September 30, 2018, the promotional film on voluntary non-remunerated blood donation acted by Chinese actor Wang Kai was released. The news that he worked as a public welfare ambassador became the hottest topic online according to the online blood public opinion monitoring in 2018 (Table 2-2). A series of publicity activities for voluntary non-remunerated blood donation, such as the 20th anniversary of the implementation of the *Law of Blood Donation* and the 2018 World Blood Donor Day, were on the top search list on social media, and the awareness of voluntary non-remunerated blood donation had become increasingly strong. See Table 2-2 for the top news of blood safety in 2018.

Table 2-2   Top-hit stories for blood safety 2018

No	Top-Hit Stories
1	Star Wang Kai became the public welfare ambassador for blood donation promotion film, spreading positive energy (Sep.30)
2	Residents lined up to donate blood when Mizhi students of Shaanxi province were attacked (Apr.28)
3	The 20th anniversary of the implementation of the *Law of Blood Donation* (Oct.1)
4	The nurse with "panda blood" in Yichun, Jiangxi province asked for leave to drive hundreds of kilometers across the province to donate blood (Aug.6)
5	Huainan, Anhui's blood-donating policeman went viral in cyber space (Aug.7)
6	World Blood Donor Day 2018 (Jun.14)
7	Release of promotional film for the 20th anniversary of the implementation of the *Law of Blood Donation* (Jun.8)
8	Breaking News! Points can be added to resident permit application for blood donation and eight other selfless acts (Mar.12)

Data source: network wide monitoring and collection of public opinions in 2018.

Chapter Two

Promotion of Voluntary Non-remunerated Blood Donation

I. Commendation Activities for Blood Donors Kept Its Momentum

China is committed to the constant improvement of the incentive mechanism for voluntary non-remunerated blood donation and has organized a nationwide commendation event for voluntary non-remunerated blood donation biennially. On December 13, 2018, National Health Commission of China, the Red Cross Society of China and the Health Bureau of the Logistics and Support Department of the Central Military Commission jointly held the 20th anniversary of the Implementation of the *Law of Blood Donation* and 2016-2017 Voluntary Non-remunerated Blood Donors Commendation Conference in Beijing, on which a large number of institutes, organizations and individuals were commended for their excellent performance in voluntary non-remunerated blood donation. Among them, 391,447 individuals were granted the Contribution Awards for Voluntary Non-remunerated Blood Donation, and 13 provinces were commended for their outstanding work, an increase of 35.9% over the prior conference.

In addition, for the blood collectors who were working hard at the front line of blood centers, National Health Commission of China, the Red Cross Society of China and the Health Bureau of the Logistics and Support Department of the Central Military Commission decided to commend 304 blood collection teams including Xidan Book Building of Beijing Red Cross Blood Center. Over the past 20 years, the majority of cadres and staff of blood centers, with a strong sense of duty and the highest awe for life, had continuously improved the quality of service, strengthened the building of blood quality and safety system, and effectively guaranteed the sustainable and healthy development of voluntary non-remunerated blood donation. Their pioneering and enterprising spirit and professional virtue of devotion would encourage more cadres and staff in blood centers to actively participate in the great cause of blood donation.

Furthermore, several provinces also took the 20th anniversary of the *Law of Blood Donation* as an opportunity to carry out various selection activities. Among them, China Blood Transfusion Association carried out the selection of "the Most Beautiful Voluntary Non-remunerated Blood Donors" "the Most Beautiful Blood Collection Team" and "the Most Beautiful Voluntary Non-remunerated Blood Donation Room", which not only improved donors' sense of satisfaction and mission but also enhanced the public awareness of voluntary non-remunerated blood donation.

II. Innovation of Incentive Mechanisms for Blood Donors

With the activities of the 20th anniversary of the *Law of Blood Donation*, blood collection and supply institutions in various provinces and cities continued to improve their service quality and optimize the service process. Some regions launched the thematic activity of "Improving the Blood Donation Experience", focusing on optimizing the service process and solving the problem of waiting in line before blood donation. Some provinces and cities explored the "Internet+ non-remunerated blood donation" to achieve "one-stop" personalized service and deliver more care and greater benefits to blood donors. Some blood centers installed microwave ovens in the blood donation rooms, and refreshments, drinks and souvenirs were also prepared for blood donors. Many blood centers also offered free Internet and TV in the blood collection room. After blood donation, in addition to the traditional telephone return visit, satisfaction survey, birthday greetings, test result notification and blood destination notification, many blood centers also carried out sympathy visits to relevant non-remunerated donors and closely interacted with blood donors like members from a big family. Furthermore, by working with the Red Cross, donors form deprived family backgrounds were assisted and blood donors' education funds were also set up. Some provinces had integrated non-remunerated blood donation into the assessment of cultural and ideological progress. By launching the "three exemption" policy (free bus, free park entrance, free registration for medical treatment), the enthusiasm of the public for blood donation was boosted and a sound climate for blood donation fostered (see Table 2-3 for other related welfare).

Table 2-3   Other related benefits for non-remunerated blood donors

Region	Benefits
Beijing	Blood donors, relatives and staff of group blood donation organizations were given priority to use blood under the same conditions
Fujian	Free biochemical physical examination, blood donation thank-you card, health guidance for blood donors An eye health service center was established to provide comprehensive eye health services for voluntary non-remunerated blood donors in Fujian province
Guizhou	Giving emergency blood donation to rare blood type donors and providing blood donation transportation subsidies
Henan	Golden Prize winners are free to enter the park during the flower fair; 50% discount for watching movies with a blood donation certificate; Discount for driving school with a blood donation certificate; free to participate in large-scale holiday entertainment activities by contacting businesses; sending holiday blessing SMS for free, holiday gifts, student fund, etc.
Hunan	Free physical examination for the winner of the national dedication award; support and care for the disadvantaged blood donors
Liaoning	Summary meeting for volunteers and rare blood groups; certificates for award-winning blood donors; caring activities at blood donation sites; purchase newspapers for excellent blood donors; free blood pressure measurements for donors, families and relatives
Tianjin	Transportation subsidy for emergency blood donation of rare blood type donors; Commemorative medals for blood donation of 50 times and 100 times; purchase newspapers for excellent blood donors; direct reimbursement of blood use expenses for donors through WeChat

Continued

Region	Benefits
Zhejiang	Priority hospital care to blood donors for use of blood; blood donor comfort, family assistance activities with the Red Cross for disadvantaged blood donors; direct reimbursement of blood expenses at the hospital, App fee reductions and exemptions; physical examination card for blood donors who won the national dedication Award
Shandong	Provide personal accident insurance for blood donors; Online fee reductions and exemptions of blood expenses and direct reimbursement at hospital

Data source: National survey on the promotion of non-remunerated blood donation.

III. The Rights and Interests of Blood Donors Better Safeguarded

For a long time, the information between blood centers and medical institutions had not been properly shared, and the policy of "non-remunerated blood donation and free blood use" had been implemented as follows: the hospital receives payment first and then the blood donor applies for a fee reductions and exemptions from the blood center with the blood donor certificate. In 2018, some regions had worked proactively to find a more direct solution by exempting donor's expenses for clinical blood use at the hospital, which better protected blood donors' rights and interests. It also solved the long-standing pain points and difficulties in the blood use process by blood donors and their direct relatives. With the resolving of these pain points such as advance payments, red tape procedures, and multiple visits for the same purpose, blood donors enjoyed more convenience. Some provinces had also formulated policies and measures such as "Management Measures for Fee Reductions and Exemptions of Non-remunerated Blood Donors' Non-local Blood Use" and "Direct Fee Reductions and Exemptions of Clinical Blood Use of Non-remunerated Blood Donors", vigorously promoted direct fee reductions and exemptions of blood use expenses which can be directly exempted in medical institutions according to the regulations. It had also been witnesses that the implementation of preferential measures for medical treatment, streamlining of fee reductions and exemptions procedures, and the prioritized blood need of blood donors, their spouses and direct relatives strengthened. Taking Zhejiang province as an example, Hangzhou realized the information-based connectivity between the provincial blood centers and the non-remunerated blood donors of the blood-using medical institutions, and carried out the "one-stop" reduction and exemption of blood using expenses in hospitals. Shaanxi province had launched policies such as the *Administrative Measures for the Fee Reductions and Exemptions of Non-local Blood Use Expenses by Non-remunerated Blood Donors in Shaanxi province* and direct fee exemptions of clinical blood use expenses of non-remunerated blood donors. It was required that all level two hospitals in the province must carry out direct reimbursement of blood expenses before the end of December 2018.

At the same time, some provinces carried out preferential policies for the non-remunerated blood donation contribution award winners to enjoy priority treatment, priority hospitalization, partial cost deduction, etc.

In addition to the free use of blood and related preferential policies for blood donors, more and more provinces began to include clinical blood expenses in the category of medical insurance for Fee Reductions and Exemptions (Table 2-4).

Table 2-4   Areas where blood expenses are included in the medical insurance for fee reductions and exemptions catalogue

Region	City
Beijing	Beijing
Tianjin	Tianjin
Shanghai	Shanghai
Chongqing	Chongqing
Anhui	Bengbu/Bozhou/Chuzhou/Huaibei
Gansu	Dingxi/Jiayuguan/Jinchang/Linxiazhou/Longnan
Guizhou	Anshun/Qianxinan/Tongren/Liupanshui
Hebei	Shijiazhuang/Qinhuangdao/Baoding/Langfang/Tangshan/Hengshui/Xingtai/Handan/Cangzhou/Zhangjiakou
Henan	Anyang/Jiaozuo/Luoyang/Puyang/Shangqiu/Xinxiang/Xuchang/Zhoukou
Hubei	Wuhan

Continued

Region	City
Hunan	Changsha/Changde/Loudi/Xiangxi/Huaihua/Shaoyang/Xiangtan/Yiyang/Yueyang/Zhuzhou
Jilin	Jilin/Yanbian/Tonghua
Jiangsu	Nanjing/Huai'an/Lianyungang/Nantong/Taizhou/Suqian/Zhenjiang
Jiangxi	Fuzhou/Ji'an/Nanchang/Jiujiang/Shangrao/Yingtan/Pingxiang
Xinjiang	Ürümqi/Hotan/Yili
Zhejiang	Ningbo/Huzhou/Jinhua/Lishui/Quzhou/Shaoxing/Wenzhou
Yunnan	Kunming/Wenshanzhou/Honghezhou/Zhaotong/Dali/Lincang/Yuxi/Baoshan/Pu'er/Chuxiong/Dehong/Xishuangbanna/Nujiang
Sichuan	Deyang/Leshan/Yibin/Chengdu/Ganzi/Aba/Ya'an/Ziyang/Panzhihua/Bazhong/Neijiang/Liangshan
Hainan	Covering the whole province
Guangdong	Guangzhou/Shenzhen/Foshan/Maoming/Shaoguan/Dongguan
Guangxi	Guilin/Hechi/Laibin/Chongzuo/Wuzhou/Beihai/Qinzhou

Data source: National survey on the promotion of non-remunerated blood donation.

Chapter Three

Voluntary Non-remunerated Blood Donation

In order to achieve the sustained development of non-remunerated blood donation, Chinese blood collection and supply institutions have attached great importance to the building of a voluntary non-remunerated blood donation team by fostering a social climate that advocates non-remunerated blood donation, and establishing a long-term mechanism for non-remunerated blood donation. At present, most cities in China have gradually established a diversified volunteer service team for non-remunerated blood donation, which had developed into a variety of affiliations to other organizations, such as the Red Cross, the Volunteers' Federation, the Lion Clubs and other civil independent legal person organizations. Many provinces and cities held regular blood donors' gatherings, and set up several squads of contingency blood donation, rare blood donation, apheresis platelet collection, etc. Some provinces and cities had established a "blood station+community" model, which not only provided office area and equipment for volunteer organizations, but also carried out mobilization activities to enhance friendship and maintain in-depth cooperation with volunteers. Some colleges and universities, social and civil organizations have set up volunteer teams for non-remunerated blood donation, by cooperating proactively with the government and relevant departments, the management of volunteer service organizations was strengthened with the sharing of volunteer resources and regular training provided. The volunteer team continued to grow in stability. All volunteers participated with great enthusiasm the publicity, recruitment and service of non-remunerated blood donation, and the work was carried out in a standardized and orderly manner. For instance, Tianjin developed a group recruitment mode, and carried out group non-remunerated blood donation. Up to now, more than 20 organizations had participated in blood donation. Since its establishment, the Nanjing Red Cross voluntary blood donation service team had registered nearly 10,000 volunteers. In 2018, the total number of volunteers reached 2,546, with a total service time of 12,864.5 hours, setting a record high. See Table 2-5 for details of the volunteer teams in various provinces and cities.

Table 2-5   Establishment of voluntary blood donation teams in all provinces (municipalities directly under the central government)

Region	City	Total number of registered volunteers	Total number of volunteer teams	Total number of volunteer service stations
Anhui	Anqing	80	3	5
	Bozhou	200	4	4
	Chizhou	635	2	4
	Lu'an	78	4	3
	Ma'anshan	276	3	6
	Wuhu	550	3	6
	Suzhou	568	1	—
Beijing	Beijing	7,135	54	41
Fujian	Fuzhou	220	20	About 50 (fixed, rural areas, colleges and universities)
	Xiamen	258	6	10
	Longyan	80	2	5
	Ningde	63	1	1
	Putian	89	1	5
	Quanzhou	235	4	16
	Sanming	3,036	1	—

Continued

Region	City	Total number of registered volunteers	Total number of volunteer teams	Total number of volunteer service stations
Gansu	Lanzhou	352	16	—
	Dingxi	300	5	16
	Jiayuguan	64	1	1
	Jinchang	50	2	2
	Longnan	38	2	2
	Pingliang	2,000	15	1
	Tianshui	162	1	9
	Wuwei	61	1	3
Guizhou	Guiyang	100	1	5
	Anshun	377	1	8
	Bijie	116	8	8
	Qianxinan	55	1	1
	Tongren	65	70	2
Hainan	Haikou	892	12	10
Hebei	Shijiazhuang	9,751	157	182
Henan	Anyang	500	3	11
	Hebi	315	3	1
	Luoyang	330	1	12
	Luohe	188	1	7
	Nanyang	346	9	18
	Pingdingshan	1,635	12	10
	Puyang	580	1	10
	Xinxiang	430	6	6
	Xinyang	804	6	2
	Xuchang	150	3	8
Heilongjiang	—	1,748	8	19
Hubei	Wuhan	1,200	55	8 (excluding colleges and universities)

Continued

Region	City	Total number of registered volunteers	Total number of volunteer teams	Total number of volunteer service stations
Hunan	Changsha	5,000	20	32
	Changde	329	3	8
	Loudi	176	1	8
	Chenzhou	237	1	1
	Hengyang	136	1	6
	Huaihua	286	4	4
	Shaoyang	220	1	1
	Xiangtan	5,264	30	10
	Yiyang	282	1	2
	Yueyang	1,400	22	8
	Zhuzhou	695	1	15
Jilin	Jilin	70	1	2
	Yanbian	126	1	1
	Songyuan	458	1	2
Jiangsu	Nanjing	1,158	1	—
	Changzhou	1,050	1	16
	Huaian	285	1	6
	Lianyungang	2,800	11	105
	Nantong	1,028	1	7
	Suzhou	169	1	5
	Taizhou	391	4	4
	Wuxi	494	7	—
	Suqian	85	1	1
	Xuzhou	2,218	9	32
	Yangzhou	1,027	5	21
	Zhenjiang	91	1	8

Continued

Region	City	Total number of registered volunteers	Total number of volunteer teams	Total number of volunteer service stations
Jiangxi	Fuzhou	1,450	5	15
	Ji'an	249	7	17
	Nanchang	98	5	8
	Jiujiang	350	7	7
	Yichun	385	2	—
	Yingtan	89	2	4
	Pingxiang	170	1	9
Liaoning	—	2,750	44	57
Shanghai	—	783	4 teams, 21 squads	7
Sichuan	Chengdu	5,794	46	67
Tianjin	—	2,538	2,334	28
Yunnan	Kunming	500	8	17
Zhejiang	Ningbo	445	12	19
	Jinhua	138	1	2
	Lishui	620	12	14
	Quzhou	225	1	2
	Shaoxing	424	5	7
	Taizhou	400	9	—
	Yiwu	150	1	1
Chongqing	—	2,050	40	40

Data source: National survey on the promotion of non-remunerated blood donation.

With the efforts in past twenty years, today, practicing volunteerism and encouraging previous blood donors to participate in the voluntary blood donation service had become a strong and unneglectable driver in pushing voluntary blood donation forward. Most provinces and cities in China had built a stable voluntary non-remunerated blood donation team that were willing to donate blood and had the know-hows in publicity and recruitment. Therefore, an ideal mode had been formed with the participation of all sectors of society to jointly promote the development of non-remunerated blood donation.

Section Three

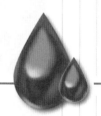

Development
and Operation
of Blood Centers

By 2018, there had been 32 blood centers, 321 regional blood banks, 99 blood banks and 1,458 fixed blood collection sites. The work force of blood centers kept growing with higher educational levels and optimized personnel structure. The infrastructure of blood centers kept improving with increased floor area. The number of fixed blood collection sites and blood transportation vehicles kept growing. Sound networking between blood centers and blood collection sites was basically in place with promoted informatization level.

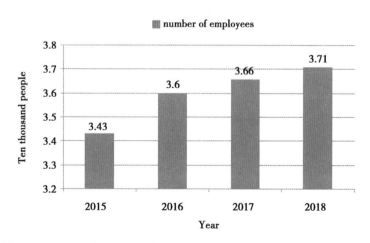

Chapter One

Employees

I. Growing Number

In 2018, employees at the Chinese blood centers totaled 37,100 (Figure 3-1), with about 16,200 employees in Eastern China, accounting for 43.67% of the total. Among the eastern region, Guangdong, Shandong and Jiangsu ranked top three in the number of employees, all of which employed more than 2,500 people. The total number in the central area was over 10,800, accounting for 29.11% of the total. The number in the western region was relatively small, and the total number of employees in the 12 provinces in the western region (autonomous regions and municipalities directly

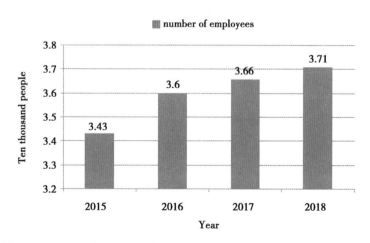

Figure 3-1   Number of employees in Chinese blood centers 2015-2018

under the central government) was over 10,100, accounting for 27.22% of the total. Xizang Zizhiqu had the smallest number of about 100 employees, followed by Qinghai and Ningxia, with only 200 respectively. Compared with the figure of 2017, the total number of employees increased by about 500 people, an increase of 1.4%. The number in eastern and western region was growing, with the largest growth in the latter, registering an increase of about 500 people, among which Guangxi and Guizhou were the top 2 provinces with an growth of around 200 and 100 people respectively. The number of employees in the central region reduced by about 180 people, and Jiangxi is where the most loss occurred, of about 200 people.

II. Higher Educational Background

In 2018, there were 116 employees with doctoral degree in Chinese blood centers, accounting for 0.32% of the total number. These doctoral employees were mainly based in the eastern and central region (except for Shanxi and Anhui), with a total number of 79 people, accounting for 68.10% of the total number of doctoral employees. In Sichuan, Chongqing, Yunnan and Shaanxi of the western region, 37 doctoral employees had been brought in with 24 of them in Shaanxi, ranking top. There were about 1,300 employees with master's degree, accounting for 3.65% of the total number of employees. The eastern region has the largest share of 56.16%. There were more than 100 employees with master's degree in Liaoning, Shandong and Jiangsu respectively. Among all the provinces (autonomous regions and municipalities directly under the central government), Beijing had the highest proportion of employees with master's degree (9.20%). The lowest number was found in Xizang Zizhiqu and Hainan (2 and 3 respectively), and the lowest proportion of employees with master's degree in relation to the total number of employees was in Hainan (1.12%). The number of employees holding a bachelor's degree was about 18,500, accounting for 51.01% of the total number of employees. Hebei, Jiangsu, Shandong, Henan and Guangdong ranked among the top, each with over 1,200 employees, and Xizang Zizhiqu had the smallest number (19); the number of employees with junior college degree or below accounted for 30.05% and 14.97% respectively (Figure 3-2). Compared with 2017, there

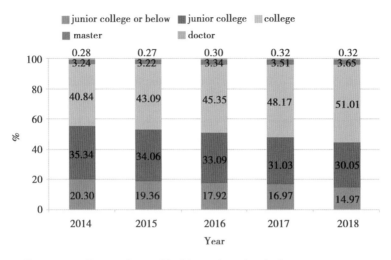

Figure 3-2 Proportions of holders of academic degrees 2014-2018

is little change in the number and proportion of doctoral employees. The proportion of master's degree holding employees has increased by 0.14%. The number of master's degree holding employees in the central and western regions was basically the same. The number of masters in the eastern region increase of 26 people, with the largest increase in Jiangsu (10ven), followed by Jilin (9). The largest decrease of master employees was witnessed in Guangxi (19), followed by Hunan (9). The proportion of bachelor degree-holding employees increased by 2.84%, with the number up by 700 people. The number in the eastern region increased by over 400 people, among which Hebei increased the most (110), followed by Jiangsu (103). Jiangxi and Guangxi witnessed the largest decrease of bachelor degree-holding employees (71 and 142 respectively). The number and proportion of employees with junior college and below degrees, had shown a general downward trend.

III. Optimizing Personnel Structure

In 2018, there were 27,200 health technicians, accounting for 73.44%. According to the *Basic Standards for Blood Centers* issued by the former Ministry of Health, health technicians in blood centers shall account for at least 75% of the total number of employees. There are 12 provinces (autonomous regions and municipalities directly under the central government) that met the requirement, including 3 in the eastern area: Tianjin, Shanghai and Zhejiang, 5 in the central area: Shanxi, Anhui, Jiangxi, Hubei and Hunan and four in the western area: Guizhou, Gansu, Qinghai and Ningxia. The highest proportion was found in Hubei (80.40%). There were 19 provinces (autonomous regions and municipalities directly under the central government) with a proportion of less than 75%, the lowest being Xizang Zizhiqu (55.88%). The health technicians were mainly registered nurses at about 13,800 people, accounting for 50.89% of the total number of health technicians. In terms of registered nurses, they mainly concentrated in the eastern region with the number exceeded 6,000, among which Jiangsu and Guangdong were the top 2. The number in the western region was relatively small at about 3,300 people. Among them, only 7 people were based in Xizang Zizhiqu, 50 were in Qinghai and 95 in Ningxia. The highest proportion of registered nurses was in Hunan (62.63%), and the lowest in Qinghai (27.78%).

There were about 7,100 inspectors, accounting for 26.22%. There were more than 3,000 in the eastern region where Jiangsu and Guangdong had the largest proportion, both had more than 500 inspectors. The total number of inspectors in the central and western regions was similar, with only 8 in Xizang Zizhiqu, 51 in Qinghai and 75 in Ningxia. The highest proportion of inspectors was in Xizang Zizhiqu (42.11%), and the lowest in Beijing (14.45%). The number of certified (Assistant) physicians and other health technicians was about 3,700 and 2,600, respectively, as was shown in Figure 3-3. Compared with 2017, the percentage of health technicians increased by 2%. The proportions of health technical personnel in 20 provinces (autonomous regions and municipalities directly under the central government) were increasing, with Qinghai and Gansu province increased the most, from 69.00% to 80.72% and 65.70% to 75.92% respectively, each experiencing an increase of more than 10 percentage points. The proportion in 11 provinces (autonomous regions and municipalities directly under the central government) were decreasing, with Shaanxi province decreased the most, from 78.81% to 73.67%, a drop of 5.14%. In addition, the overall proportion of registered nurses and inspectors was increasing, and the proportions of certified (Assistant) physicians and other health technicians were decreasing.

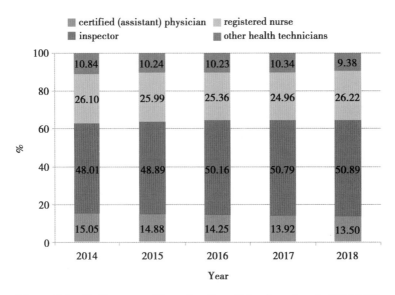

Figure 3-3   Staff composition of national blood centers in 2014-2018

In 2018, there were about 28,800 employees with professional titles in the blood center industry, accounting for 77.70%. Among them, senior, intermediate and junior titles accounted for 12.56%, 29.67% and 57.77% respectively (Figure 3-4). The number of employees with senior professional title was the largest in the eastern region, at about 1,600 people, accounting for 46.80% of the total number of senior professional

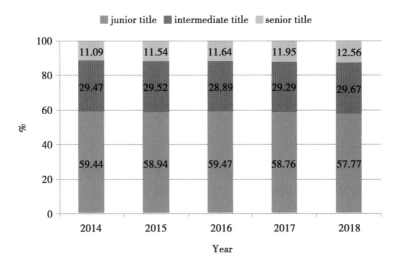

Figure 3-4   Professional titles of employees 2014-2018

title holders. The number of senior professional title holders was basically the same in the central and western region. The highest proportion of senior professional titles was found in Nei Mongol Zizhiqu (25.99%), the lowest in Anhui (3.76%), followed by Hainan (4.95%). The number of intermediate professional titles in the eastern region reached around 4,000 people, accounting for 48.05% of the total number of intermediate professional title holders, and the proportion in the central region was 7% higher than that in the western region. The highest proportion of intermediate professional titles was found in Tianjin (41.72%) and the lowest in Xinjiang (19.15%), followed by Ningxia (20.90%). The number of junior professional titles in the eastern region is about 7,000, accounting for 43.23% of the total number of junior professional title holders. The number in the central and western region was basically the same. The proportion of junior professional titles was the highest in Xinjiang (69.71%) and the lowest in Tianjin (45.09%), followed by Heilongjiang (48.11%). Compared with 2017, the proportion of employees with professional titles increased by 1.70%, the proportion of intermediate and senior professional titles respectively witnessed an increase of 0.38% and 0.61%, whereas the proportion of junior professional titles decreased from 58.76% to 57.77%. The number of employees with senior, intermediate and junior professional titles in the east remained basically the same. The number of employees with senior and intermediate titles in the central region had increased by about 100 people, while the number of employees with junior titles had slightly decreased. The number of employees with senior, intermediate and junior professional titles in the western region had increased by over 300 people in total. The number of senior titles increased by the largest margin in Jiangsu (36); The number of intermediate titles increased the most in Anhui (44); The number of junior titles increased the most in Jilin (92); The number of senior titles decreased the most in Hebei (10) and the number of intermediate and junior titles decreased the most in Guangxi (49 and 190 respectively).

Chapter Two

Infrastructure

I. Continuous Growth of Floor Area

In 2018, the national blood centers covered an area of 2.16 million m^2 and a building area of 2.09 million m^2 respectively (Figure 3-5). The eastern, central and western regions respectively covered an area of about 800,000 m^2, 70,000 m^2 and 600,000 m^2. 6 provinces (autonomous regions and municipalities directly under the central government) each had covered an area of more than 100,000 m^2, among which the largest was Henan, reaching 177,000 m^2. The smallest was in Xizang Zizhiqu

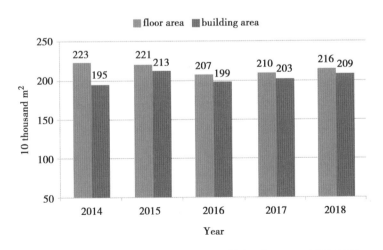

Figure 3-5   Floor and building area of blood centers 2014-2018

with only 5,200 m^2. The building area in the eastern region was about 920,000 m^2, and that in the central region was about 600,000 m^2, about 30,000 m^2 more than that in the western region. The largest building area was found in Jiangsu (223,500 m^2), and the smallest was in Xizang Zizhiqu (3,700 m^2). Compared with 2017, the floor area and building area increased by 2.70% and 2.90% respectively. There were 8 provinces (autonomous regions and municipalities directly under the central government) and 10 provinces (autonomous regions and municipalities directly under the central government) that had experienced an increase of their floor area and building area, whereas 13 and 12 had witnessed a decline of their floor area and building area. Jiangsu had increased the most in terms of floor area and building area, up by 25,300 and 31,200 m^2 respectively. Guangxi experienced the biggest decline of floor and building areas, down by 16,100 and 32,300 m^2 respectively.

II. Continuous Improvement of Construction

According to incomplete statistics, 37 blood centers had chosen new sites for construction from 2014 to 2018, involving 17 provinces (autonomous regions and municipalities directly under the central government). Covering an area of 125,100 m^2 before construction, it had been expected that after construction the floor space would reach 334,700 m^2, an increase of 209,600 m^2, up by 167.55%. A total of 15 blood stations had been reconstructed on the original sites, involving 10 provinces (autonomous regions and municipality directly under the central government). Prior to the reconstruction, the sites covered an area of 71,800 m^2, and after reconstruction the number become 126,900 m^2, witnessing an increase of 55,100 square meters, up by 76.74%. A total of 18 blood centers had finished construction, involving 7 provinces (autonomous regions and municipalities directly under the central government). The covered area before construction was 71,400 m^2, and after construction was 204,100 m^2, an increase of 132,700 m^2, up by 185.85%, see Figure 3-6 for details.

III. Continuous Improvement of Infrastructure

The number of fixed blood collection sites were an important

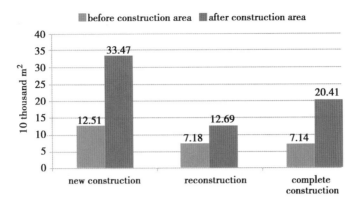

Figure 3-6   Construction of national blood centers in 2014-2018

indicator for blood collection capacity while that of blood collection and transportation vehicles was a great benchmark for service capacity. In 2018, there were 1,458 fixed blood collection sites, 1,583 blood collection vehicles and 1,483 blood transportation vehicles in China (Figure 3-7). Fixed blood collection sites were mainly concentrated in the eastern region (597), among which Jiangsu and Guangdong had 113 and 112 respectively, ranking top two. Hainan had only one fixed blood collection site while Tianjin and Beijing each had 2. In the central region, there were 461 fixed

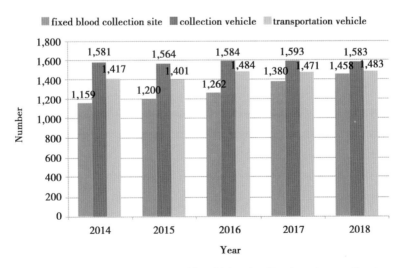

Figure 3-7   National numbers of fixed blood collection sites, collection vehicles and transportation vehicles 2014-2018

blood collection sites, among which Henan and Hunan were the top two, registering 97 and 92 respectively. Jilin and Heilongjiang were at the end of the row, having 39 and 30 respectively; In the western region, there were 400 fixed blood collection sites, with 95 in Sichuan and 56 in Chongqing, which both ranked among the top. There were 6 fixed blood collection sites in Qinghai and none in Xizang Zizhiqu. There were 711 blood collection vehicles in the eastern region, accounting for 45% of the total. The number of blood collection vehicles in Jiangsu, Shandong and Guangdong ranked the top three, all of which exceeded 110. Hainan had the smallest number (7), and the central region had 20 more vehicles than the western region. The eastern region had 598 blood transportation vehicles, the largest amount compared with 462 in the western region and 423 in the central region. In the eastern part, Guangdong had the largest number of blood transportation vehicles (117), followed by Jiangsu (99). In the western region, Sichuan had the most blood transportation vehicles (82). In the central part, Henan had the largest number (81). Xizang Zizhiqu, Tianjin and Ningxia had smaller numbers, only 2, 8 and 11 respectively. Compared with 2017, the number of fixed blood collection sites saw an increase of 78 sets, up by 5.65%. The number of blood collection vehicles experienced a decrease of 10 sets, down by 0.63%. The number of blood transportation vehicles witnessed an increase of 12 sets, up by 0.82%. In terms of fixed blood collection sites, Liaoning and Zhejiang in the eastern region each lessened by 1 site, Shanghai and Hainan remained unchanged, and all the other provinces (autonomous regions and municipalities directly under the central government) had experienced an increase, with Fujian increased the most (23), followed by Shandong (6). Shanxi and Henan in the central area did not change in the number of fixed blood collection sites, with Heilongjiang and Anhui saw a decrease by 2 and 1 respectively and the rest central provinces witnessing an increase. Among them, Hubei increased the most (4). In the western region, Nei Mongol Zizhiqu and Guangxi decreased by 2 and 3 respectively, with Guizhou remained mostly the same. Xizang Zizhiqu still had no fixed blood collection site, while the numbers for all the rest increased. Among them, Yunnan increased the most (9). In terms of blood collection vehicles, the number in 12 provinces (as well as autonomous regions and municipalities directly under the central government) were increasing, with Jiangsu province increased the most (11), and 11 provinces (as well as autonomous regions and municipalities directly under the central government) decreased, and Hubei province had the largest decrease (12). The number of blood transportation vehicles in 12 provinces (as well as autonomous regions and municipalities directly under the central government) was increasing, with Zhejiang increased the most (8), and 7 provinces (as well as autonomous regions and municipalities directly under the central government) decreased, with Jiangxi and Guangdong province decreased the most, 26 and 22 respectively.

Chapter Three

Informatization Building

I. Sound Networking among Blood Centers

Apart from Shandong, Shaanxi, Qinghai and Xizang Zizhiqu, all the other 26 provinces (as well as autonomous regions and municipalities directly under the central government) had realized the information-based management of blood centers. According to research, the blood centers had all realized the networking between themselves and the blood collection sites. In terms of the networking between blood centers, 12 provinces (as well as autonomous regions, municipalities directly under the central government) had realized the complete networking within their respective jurisdiction; 7 provinces (as well as autonomous regions and municipalities directly under the central government) were partially networked; and 7 provinces (as well as autonomous regions, and municipalities directly under the central government) were not networked. In terms of the networking between blood centers and hospitals, 4 provinces (as well as autonomous regions and municipalities directly under the central government) had realized complete networking within their respective jurisdiction, 15 provinces (as well as autonomous regions and municipalities directly under the central government) were partially networked, and 7 provinces (as well as autonomous regions, and municipalities directly under the central government) were not networked. In terms of the networking between blood centers and provincial health administrative departments, 14 provinces (as well as autonomous regions and municipalities directly under the central government) had realized complete networking, 4 provinces (as well as autonomous regions and municipalities directly under the central government) were partially networked, and 8 provinces (as well as autonomous regions and municipalities directly under the central government) were not networked. Beijing, Shanghai, Hebei and Jiangxi all adopted the 4 mentioned modes, accounting for 15.38% of the total.

Table 3-1   Informatization building of blood centers in 2018

Function	Complete	Partial	Realization
Networking between blood centers	12 (46%)	7 (27%)	7 (27%)
Networking between blood centers and hospitals	4 (15%)	15 (58%)	7 (27%)
Networking blood centers with provincial health administrative departments	14 (54%)	4 (15%)	8 (31%)

II. Continuous Innovation of Information Management Mode

In 2018, on the basis of information-based networking, some regions in China continued to explore innovative working modes. Hubei province initiated the "Internet+" blood management, and built an integrated management platform which integrated non-remunerated blood donors service management platform, clinical blood support platform, blood contingency command platform, blood information management platform and blood donation education base. Hebei province provided information support for the arrangement and deployment of the blood management system through the real-time analyses of 17 management indicators from 7 major categories, such as blood collection and supply volume, blood donation rate per thousand population, and the building of emergency blood donation team. Guangxi had built a blood management application system including blood collection and supply information, dynamic early warning and monitoring of blood inventory, blood distribution, fee reductions and exemptions for blood use in other places, so as to realize the whole process management of "from blood vessel to blood management" (a pun in Chinese language). Zhejiang Blood Cloud Platform had realized sound connectivity with the Provincial and Municipal Health and Family Planning Commission, almost all the blood centers and blood banks in Zhejiang province (except for the ones in Wenzhou city), provincial hospitals in Hangzhou, municipal hospitals and municipal donation management centers, etc. At the same time, the upgrade of blood management information system was carried out throughout the province. The Shanghai Integrated Management Platform for Clinical Blood Use had realized connectivity and information sharing among the blood management institutions, blood collection and supply institutions and hospitals in the city, as well as the blood information networking in the Jiangsu, Zhejiang and Shanghai region.

Section Four

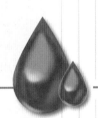

The Recruitment
of Blood Donors
and Blood
Collection

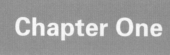

Chapter One

Blood Donation Types

In order to further refine the working mode of non-remunerated blood donation and improve the safety of blood donation in China, mutual-aid blood donation system was completely abolished in 2018. At various localities and authorities, the strengthening of the service capacity of non-remunerated blood donation and the promotion of group voluntary non-remunerated blood donation have managed to cater to the fluctuations of the demand for blood in clinical use. On the one hand, it is important to improve the mobilization and promotion of non-remunerated blood donation and increase blood stations as well as build up the capabilities of promoting voluntary non-remunerated blood donations. On the other hand, bolstering the promotion of group donations effectively solves the problem of insufficient donations during the off-season, as well as the inadequate supply of rare blood types or blood for contingency use. So far, China has gradually developed a balanced approach that combines individual and group voluntary non-remunerated blood donations.

From 2014 to 2018, the total amount of donated blood and the number of blood donors continuously broke new records, and the ratio of group voluntary non-remunerated blood donations grew from 20.7% to 27.2% (Figure 4-1).

In 2018, the total number of individual voluntary non-remunerated blood donors in China was 10.676 million, up 1.7% over 2017. In this mix,

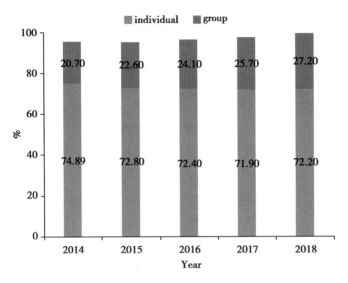

Figure 4-1   Percentage of individual and group voluntary
non-remunerated blood donations, 2014-2018

individual whole blood donation occurred 9.636 million times, up 0.7%
over 2017, and platelet donation occurred 1.04 million times, up 12.5% over
2017 (Table 4-1).

Table 4-1   Number and growth of individual voluntary
non-remunerated blood donation, 2014–2018

Year	Donation/ 10 thousand people	Growth/ %	Whole Blood/10 thousand people	Growth/ %	Platelet/ 10 thousand people	Growth/ %
2014	970.8	—	897.3	—	73.5	—
2015	961.3	–1.0	881.9	–1.7	79.4	8.0
2016	1,013.1	5.4	927.6	5.2	85.5	7.7
2017	1,049.4	3.6	957.0	3.2	92.4	8.1
2018	1,067.6	1.7	963.6	0.7	104.0	12.5

In 2018, the total number of group voluntary non-remunerated blood
donations in China was 4.027 million person-times, representing an
increase of 7.4% over 2017(Table 4-2).

Table 4-2   Number and growth of group voluntary
non-remunerated blood donations, 2014–2018

Year	Donation/10 thousand people	Growth/%	Whole Blood/10 thousand people	Growth/%	Platelet/10 thousand people	Growth/%
2014	268.3	—	265.8	—	2.5	—
2015	298.5	11.3	296.0	11.3	2.6	3.1
2016	337.2	13.0	334.5	13.0	2.7	4.8
2017	375.2	11.2	372.3	11.3	2.8	5.5
2018	402.7	7.4	399.1	7.2	3.6	25.8

Regional differences in the ratio and distribution of group voluntary non-remunerated blood donations could be observed clearly (Figure 4-2). Group voluntary non-remunerated blood donations ratio was more than 45% in Shanghai and Zhejiang province but less than 15% in Tianjin municipality, the Nei Mongol Zizhiqu, Hubei province and the Xinjiang Production and Construction Corps.

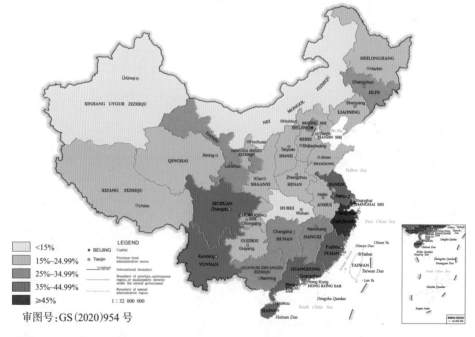

审图号：GS（2020）954 号

Figure 4-2   Distribution of group voluntary non-remunerated blood donation in 2018 (Remark: the data of this figure do not include HONG KONG SAR, MACAU SAR and TAIWAN Province.)

Chapter Two

Donor Backgrounds

The gender structure of donors in China evolved on a balanced basis. The ratio of female donors rose year by year (Figure 4-3).

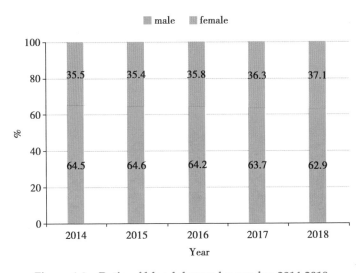

Figure 4-3   Ratio of blood donors by gender, 2014-2018

Most of the donors aged between 18 and 45. In 2018, donors in this age-group accounted for nearly 77.5% of the total. From 2014 to 2018, nearly 770,000 donors aged over 55 donated their blood. The ratio of donors aged between 26 and 44 shrank, while the ratio of donors aged between 45 and 55 rose (Figure 4-4).

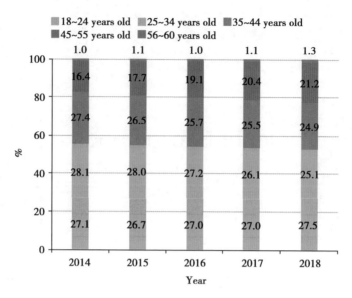

Figure 4-4　Ratio of blood donors by age, 2014-2018

The highest diplomas of donors were primarily from middle-school, high-school and junior college. The ratio of donors with a bachelor's degree increased from 16.2% in 2014 to 19.8% in 2018 (Figure 4-5).

Donors were students, office clerks, farmers, workers, medical staff, civil servants, teachers, military personnel and workers of other trades (eg.

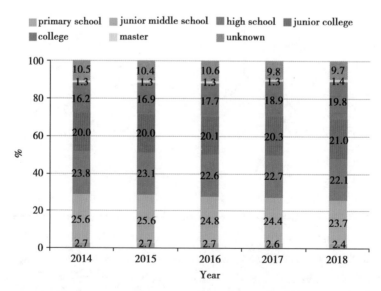

Figure 4-5　Ratio of blood donors by educational background, 2014-2018

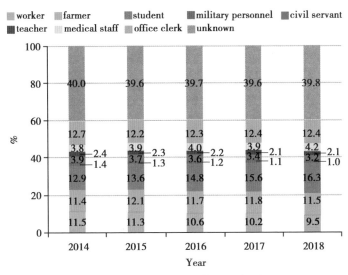

Figure 4-6   Ratio of blood donors by profession, 2014-2018

freelancers). In 2018, college students accounted for 16.3% of the total mix of donors, up 0.7 percentage points over the previous year (Figure 4-6).

In 2018, civil servants, college students and medical staff across the country set a good example in voluntary non-remunerated blood donation. The blood donation per 1,000 civil servants, college students and medical staff personnel was 66.6, 89.5 and 55.5, respectively, much higher than the average national blood donation rate per 1,000 people, which was 11.1 (Figure 4-7).

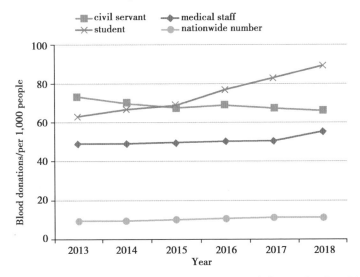

Figure 4-7   Number of blood donations per 1,000 people by profession, 2014-2018

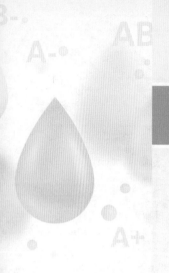

Chapter Three

Blood Collection

The blood donation rate per 1,000 people is a key indicator in evaluating the blood supply performance of a country or a region. In 2018, China's national blood donation rate was 11.1 per 1,000. The blood donation rate exceeded 12 per 1,000 in Beijing municipality, Shanghai municipality, Jiangsu province, Zhejiang province, Henan province, Shanxi province and Tianjin municipality, whereas in the Xizang Zizhiqu and some other provinces the blood donation rate was less than 6 per 1,000 (Figure 4-8). The annual trends indicate that China's blood donation rate per 1,000 people increased gradually from 2014 to 2018. The donation rate in 2018 was 2.9 percentage points higher than that of 2017 (Figure 4-9).

Since 1998, the volume of voluntary non-remunerated blood donations nationwide has witnessed growth for nearly twenty consecutive years. Against the backdrop of completely abolishing the mutual-aid blood donation law, total blood donation and the number of blood donors still grew. In 2018, 14.79 million blood donations were collected, up by 1.4% compared with 2017, of which there were 13.7 million whole blood donations, up by 0.9% over 2017, and 1.09 million platelet donations, up by 6.8% over 2017 (Figure 4-10).

Growth momentum was maintained in the volume of blood collected nationwide from 2014 to 2018. In 2018, 23.28 million units of whole blood and 1.78 million units of platelets were collected, up by 0.4% and 10.9%

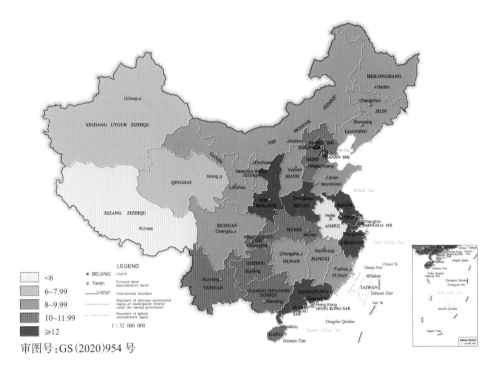

审图号：GS（2020）954 号

Figure 4-8   Distribution of blood donations per 1,000 people in 2018
（Remark: the data of this figure do not include HONG KONG SAR, MACAU SAR and
TAIWAN Province.）

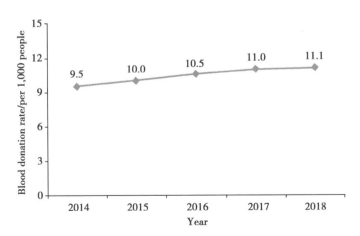

Figure 4-9   Blood donation rate per 1,000 people, 2014-2018

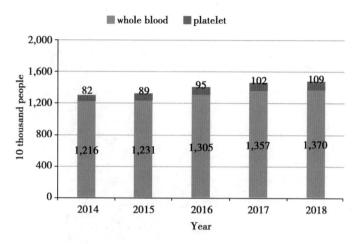

Figure 4-10   Number of blood donations, 2014-2018

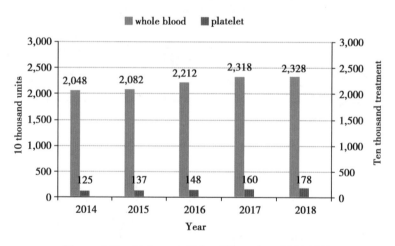

Figure 4-11   Volume of blood donation, 2014-2018

compared with 2017, respectively (Figure 4-11).

The *Law of Blood Donation* stipulates that the volume of blood collected per donor per donation shall be around 200ml and must not exceed 400ml. In 2018, the donation of 200ml of blood per donation accounted for 18.4%. The average volume of blood donated was 340.4ml, a drop of 0.1ml from 2017 (Figure 4-12).

Confidential unit exdusion (CUE) refers to the situation when, due to a donor's high-risk behavior (including 1. having multiple sexual partners,

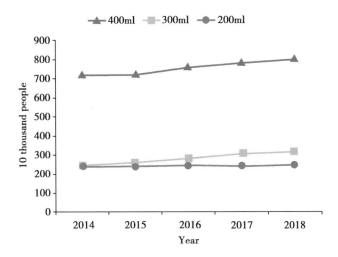

Figure 4-12   Number of whole blood donations by volume, 2014-2018

2. working as a sex worker/prostitute, 3. homosexuality, 4. drug use via injection, 5. engaging in tattooing or ritual blood-letting, and 6. having sex with any of the above-mentioned people) that might have contaminated the donated blood, the national blood service is informed after donation not to use the donated blood for clinical purposes. In accordance with the regulations, the national blood service shall, on the basis of protecting the privacy of the donor, label the blood as unqualified confidential blood. Properly conducting the confidential withdrawal of blood from donors engaging in high-risk behavior can further guarantee the level of blood safety and can greatly reduce the occurrence of the "window period" of transfusion-transmitted diseases. Growth momentum has been maintained in the national efforts towards the confidential withdrawal of blood from donors engaging in high-risk behavior since 2016. In 2018, the total volume of confidentially withdrawn blood in China was 5,297.4U, up 53.2% over 2017 (Figure 4-13).

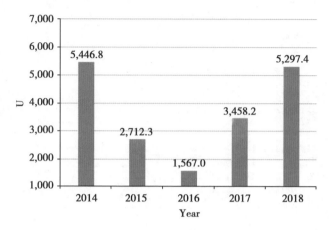

Figure 4-13   Volume of confidentially withdrawn blood, 2014-2018

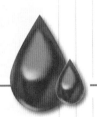

Blood Testing and Quality Assurance

Chapter One

Blood Testing at Blood Centers

I. Pre-donation Blood Screening

Pre-donation blood screening enables some ineligible donors to refrain from donation, effectively reducing discarded donations and the waste of resources. This is an important measure to ensure blood quality. At present, hemoglobin (Hb), alanine aminotransferase (ALT), hepatitis B virus surface antigen (HBsAg), the ABO blood group, erythrocyte volume and platelet count are the main screening methods. With the continuous improvement of health consultation and the physical examination of blood donors, the rate of ineligible blood donations in pre-donation screening is decreasing (Figure 5-1).

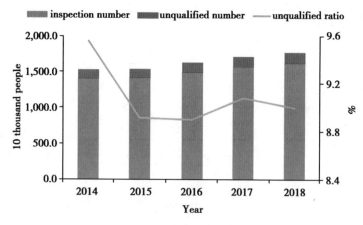

Figure 5-1   Number of ineligible blood donations in blood screening, 2014-2018

In 2018, the main areas with a high ineligibility rate in the pre-donation blood tests were the Xizang Zizhiqu, Qinghai province and Ningxia Huizu Zizhiqu. The ineligibility rate of pre-donation rapid screening in these areas exceeded 14%, while in Hunan and Hubei provinces these figures were all below 6% (Figure 5-2).

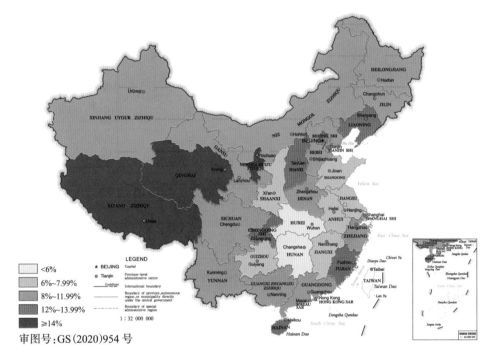

审图号：GS（2020）954 号

Figure 5-2   Distribution of the rate of ineligible blood donations in
pre-donation screening in 2018

（Remark: the data of this figure do not include HONG KONG SAR, MACAU SAR and TAIWAN Province.）

In 2018 pre-donation screenings, the incidence of HBsAg non-conformities decreased 6.3% compared to 2017, while the incidence of ALT and Hb non-conformities increased 3.8% and 2.6%, respectively, compared to 2017 (Figure 5-3).

The main cause for ineligibility in the pre-donation screening in 2018 was ALT, accounting for 56.5% of the total, an increase of 0.3 percentage points over that of 2017. The percentage of HBsAg non-conformities was 9.7%, one percentage point less than that of 2017, and the percentage of Hb

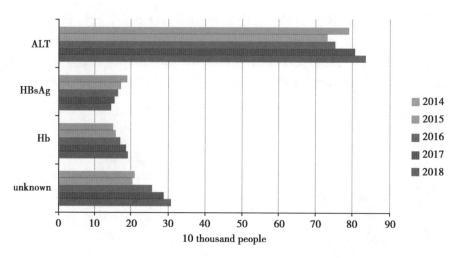

Figure 5-3　Incidence of ineligible blood donations by
pre-donation screening items, 2014-2018

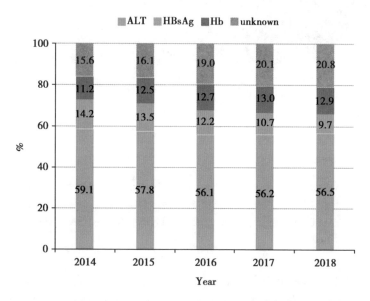

Figure 5-4　Ratio of ineligible blood donations by
pre-donation screening methods, 2014-2018

non-conformities was 12.9%, a decrease of 0.1 percentage points over that
of 2017 (Figure 5-4).

Based on the annual trends of each method tested, ineligibility due
to ALT non-conformities decreased significantly from 2014 to 2018.

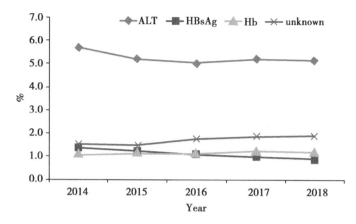

Figure 5-5   Rate of ineligible blood donations by
pre-donation screening methods, 2014-2018

Ineligibility due to HBsAg non-conformities also dropped, while that of
Hb non-conformities rose slightly (Figure 5-5).

II. Blood Laboratory Testing at Blood Centers

The tests in blood centers mainly target infectious diseases in
transfusion, including ALT, HBsAg, hepatitis C virus antibody (anti-HCV),
human immunodeficiency virus antibody (anti-HIV), Treponema pallidum
antibody (anti-TP) and nucleic acid testing (NAT). With improved blood
donor health examinations and blood pre-donation testing, the rate of
ineligible blood donations based on laboratory testing at blood centers has
declined year after year (Figure 5-6).

Laboratory testing results per 10,000 people differed from region to
region because of the differences in the incidence of epidemic infectious
diseases, the sensitivity of reagents, the setting of grey areas and the
elimination rules of blood laboratories at blood centers. Among the
provinces (as well as autonomous regions and municipalities directly
under the central government), Xizang Zizhiqu had the highest rate of
non-conformity in the laboratory testing of donated blood at blood centers
in 2018 ($\geqslant$4%) (Figure 5-7).

In 2018, the biggest cause for failing laboratory blood tests at blood
centers in China was ALT non-conformities, accounting for 39.6% of the
total. This was followed by HBsAg non-conformities, 19.1% of the total

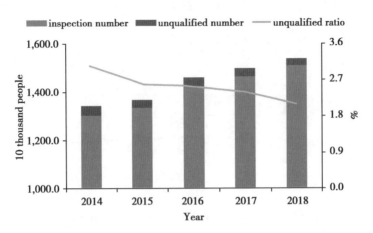

Figure 5-6   Ineligible blood donations based on
laboratory testing at blood centers, 2014-2018

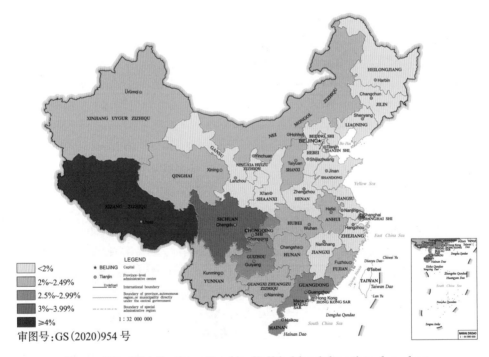

审图号:GS(2020)954号

Figure 5-7   Distribution rate of ineligible blood donations based on
laboratory testing at blood centers in 2018
(Remark: the data of this figure do not include HONG KONG SAR, MACAU SAR and
TAIWAN Province.)

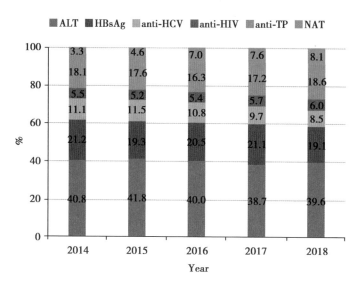

Figure 5-8   Composition of ineligible blood donations by
laboratory testing at blood centers, 2014-2018

(Figure 5-8).

From the annual data for non-conformity rates of various causes, the
percentage of ALT-caused ineligibility showed a significant downward
trend (Figure 5-9).

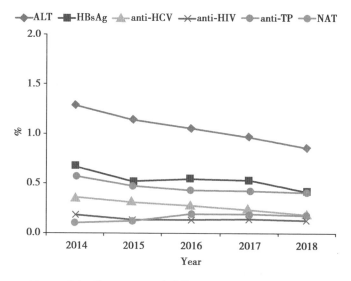

Figure 5-9   Percentage of different ineligibility causes
based on laboratory testing at blood centers, 2014-2018

The surveillance of the human T Lymphovirus (HTLV) antibody among blood donors has been carried out in China since 2016. This surveillance included all donors in Guangdong, Zhejiang and Fujian provinces. The other provinces were sampled and monitored via the random sampling of 10% of the total blood donors in their own provinces. In 2018, a total of 343,400 people were monitored in Fujian province, with 269 positive cases in primary screening, 69 of which were confirmed, for a positive conformation rate of 2.01 per 10,000. In Zhejiang province, a total of 711,000 blood samples were screened, with 109 positive results in the primary screening, though no confirmation tests were carried out. A total of 861,600 blood donors were monitored in Guangdong province, with 277 positive cases in primary screening, 13 of which were confirmed, for a positive conformation rate of 0.15 per 10,000. Among the other provinces (as well as autonomous regions and municipalities directly under the central government) that carried out sampling surveillance, 24 of them gave feedback data. With a total of 1.049 million people monitored, 14 cases were confirmed positive, for a positive conformation rate of 13 per 10,000 (Table 5-1).

Table 5-1   HTLV surveillance at blood centers, 2016-2018

Year	Blood Center/n	Screening/10 thousand	Reactive rate to screening/10 thousand	Confirmatory Positive rate/10 thousand
2016	138	250.4	4.51	0.61
2017	113	247.2	5.06	0.72
2018	94	296.5	4.06	0.55

Chapter Two

External Quality Assessment of Laboratories

I. External Quality Assessment of Laboratories for Blood Testing

(I) The EQA-based Quality Assurance program was Gradually Improved

With the upgrade of blood testing technology and the increasing number of test items, the EQA of blood collection and supply from hospitals in China was born and flourished, and it developed as a program involving multiple test items covering every aspect. In addition, its reporting has moved from newspapers to online outlets. At last, China has built an EQA-based quality assurance system. The current EQA program of the Clinical Laboratory Center of the National Health Commission (hereinafter referred to as the Clinical Laboratory Center) covers a total of 11 items in 4 quality evaluation schemes for the laboratories and institutions that collect and supply blood, including routine tests. In this way, blood safety has been ensured. The items included in each EQA scheme differ according to the different quality assurance programs selected by each blood center, hospital, reagent manufacturer or plasma center/biological products factory (Table 5-2).

(II) The Number of Institutions Participating in the EQA Program is Stable

In 2018, the laboratories of 429 blood collection and supply institutions participated in the EQA program for infectious diseases blood testing, 1,188 laboratories (including hospitals) participated in the program for blood

Table 5-2   Basic situation of the EQA schemes of laboratories

Name	Tests for	Participants			
		Category	2016/n	2017/n	2018/n
Test for Infectious Diseases	ALT/ HBsAg/anti-HCV/anti-HIV/anti-TP	Department of blood laboratory of blood center	376	366	355
		Department of quality control of blood center/ other lab	11	9	14
		Plasmapheresis center/ Biological products factory	40	40	60
Test for Blood Group	Group ABO/ Group Rh(D)	Department of blood laboratory of blood center	393	354	345
		Department of blood transfusion /Blood laboratory of medical institutions	773	785	778
		Third party inspection agency	—	43	65
Nucleic Acid Test for Viruses	HBV DNA, HCV RNA, HIV RNA	Department of blood laboratory of blood center	217	333	307
		Reagent manufacturer	9	6	6
Test for HTLV	anti-HTLV	Department of blood laboratory of blood center	—	83	81
		Biological products factory	—	1	0
		Third party inspection agency	—	2	1
		Reagent manufacturer	—	3	2

group testing, 313 participated in the program for viral nucleic acid tests, and 84 participated in tests for anti-HTLV. On a whole, the number of blood collection and supply institutions participating in the EQA programs was more stable (Figure 5-10).

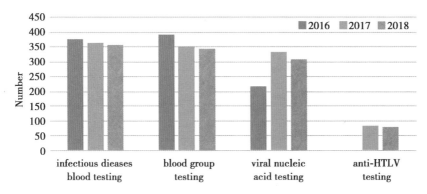

Figure 5-10   Number of laboratories participating in the EQA program of
the Clinical Laboratory Center, 2016-2018

(III) The Performance of the EQA Program Remained Stable

The EQA program for infectious diseases blood testing: 368 participating laboratories from blood centers (including some quality control departments) were asked to participate in three EQA schemes throughout the year. The overall conformity rate was good. According to the rule that the grades of the 3 quality evaluations should all be above 80 points, 350 laboratories were qualified with a qualification rate of 95.11%.

The EQA program for blood group testing: the 2018 program was changed to be conducted twice a year. A total of 371 blood centers (including the regional blood bank) participated in the program, including ABO forward typing and reverse typing and RhD blood group testing each time. There were 363 laboratories qualified for the forward typing tests for ABO, 359 for the reverse typing tests for ABO, and 364 for the RhD tests. On the whole, 358 laboratories passed the entire 2018 EQA program, with a qualification rate of 96.50%.

The EQA program for viral nucleic acid testing: there were 310 participants in the program in 2018, of which 259 were all correct, accounting for 83.55% of all blood center laboratories; additionally, 304 scored above 80 points in the two quality assessments, accounting for 98.06% of all laboratories. This was conducted in two ways: pooled testing and individual donor testing, with the former used by 274 laboratories and the latter used by 65 laboratories.

The EQA for anti-HTLV testing: there were 78 participants in 2018, 75 of which were all correct, for a qualification rate of 96.15%.

II. The EQA Program for Blood Transfusion Compatibility

(I) The Number of Institutions Participating in the EQA Program has Increased Year by Year

The 2018 EQA program included five test items: ABO forward typing, ABO reverse typing, the RhD, antibody, screening and cross-matching, and all of them have been approved by the China National Accreditation Service for Conformity Assessment (CNAS) according to the ISO/IEC 17043 standard. The participants mainly included departments for blood transfusion, laboratory departments, blood collection and supply institutions, reagent manufacturers and the blood transfusion departments and blood centers of military medical institutions. The number of participating institutions surged from 200 in 2008 to 2,144 in 2018, including 1,134 tertiary A hospitals, 465 secondary A hospitals, another 276 tertiary hospitals, 45 other secondary hospitals and 109 other hospitals. There were also 64 blood centers, 9 reagent manufacturers and 42 other institutions. The number of participants experienced rapid growth from 2008 to 2014, with an average growth rate of 39.15%. Since 2015, this number has been growing steadily, with an average growth rate of 6.93% (Figure 5-11). Currently, the EQA program covers 31 provinces (as well as autonomous regions and municipalities directly under the central government) (Figure 5-12).

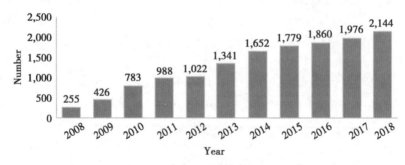

Figure 5-11   Number of institutions participating in EQA for blood
transfusion compatibility testing, 2008-2018

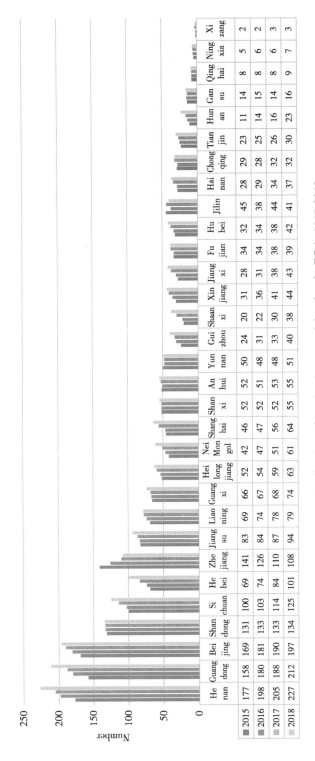

	2015	2016	2017	2018
He nan	177	198	205	227
Guang dong	158	180	188	212
Bei jing	169	181	190	197
Shan dong	131	133	133	134
Si chuan	100	103	114	125
He bei	69	74	84	101
Zhe jiang	141	126	110	108
Jiang su	83	84	87	94
Liao ning	69	74	78	79
Guang xi	66	67	68	74
Hei long jiang	52	54	59	63
Nei Mon gol	42	47	51	61
Shang hai	46	47	56	64
Shan xi	52	52	52	55
An hui	52	51	53	55
Yun nan	50	48	48	51
Gui zhou	24	31	33	40
Shaan xi	20	22	30	38
Xin jiang	31	36	41	44
Jiang xi	28	31	38	43
Fu jian	34	34	38	39
Hu bei	32	34	38	42
Jilin	45	38	44	41
Hai nan	28	29	34	37
Chong qing	29	28	32	32
Tian jin	23	25	26	30
Hun an	11	14	16	23
Gan su	14	15	14	16
Qing hai	8	8	8	9
Ning xia	5	6	6	7
Xi zang	2	2	3	3

Figure 5-12　Distribution of institutions participating in EQA, 2015-2018

(II) The Performance of the EQA Program Remained Stable

3 batches of quality assessments are carried out every year for the EQA program for blood transfusion compatibility testing, including the five items consisting of ABO forward typing, ABO reverse typing, the RhD blood group, antibody screening and cross-matching. In 2018, the quality assessment results of all participating units were qualified. See Figures 5-13 to 5-17 for the quality assessment results of each test of the EQA. See Figure 5-18 for the qualification rate of the participating institutions of all provinces (as well as autonomous regions and municipalities directly under the central government) from 2015 to 2018.

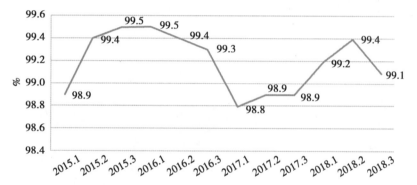

Figure 5-13   Test results for ABO forward typing, 2015-2018

Note: 2015.1 represents the first batch of the EQA program for 2015, and so on (the following figures use the same terminology).

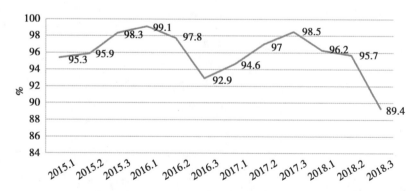

Figure 5-14   Test results for ABO reverse typing, 2015-2018

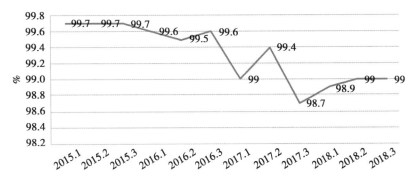

Figure 5-15　Test results for the RhD blood group, 2015-2018

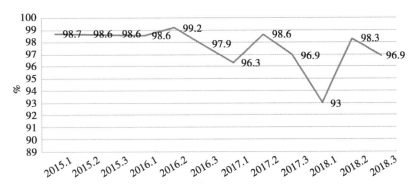

Figure 5-16　Test results for antibody screening, 2015-2018

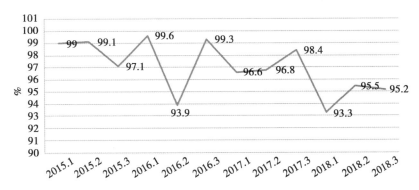

Figure 5-17　Test results for cross-matching, 2015-2018

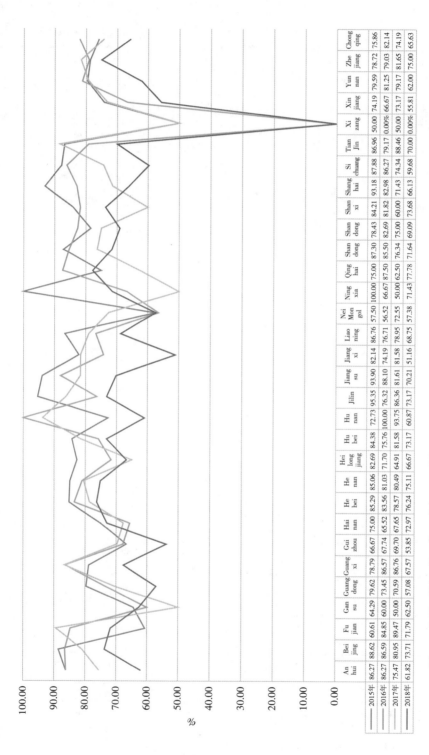

Figure 5-18 Distribution of the qualification rate for participating institutions in all five tests, 2015-2018

	An hui	Bei jing	Fu jian	Gan su	Guang dong	Guang xi	Gui zhou	Hai nan	He bei	He nan	Hei long jiang	Hu bei	Hu nan	Jilin	Jiang su	Jiang xi	Liao ning	Nei Mon gol	Ning xia	Qing hai	Shan dong	Shan xi	Shaan xi	Shang hai	Si chuang	Tian Jin	Xi zang	Xin jiang	Yun nan	Zhe jiang	Chong qing
2015年	86.27	88.62	60.61	64.29	79.62	78.79	66.67	75.00	85.29	85.06	82.69	84.38	72.73	95.35	93.90	82.14	86.76	57.50	100.00	75.00	87.30	84.21	78.43	93.18	87.88	86.96	50.00	74.19	79.59	78.72	75.86
2016年	86.27	86.59	84.85	60.00	73.45	86.57	67.74	65.52	83.56	81.03	71.70	75.76	100.00	76.32	88.10	74.19	76.71	56.52	66.67	87.50	85.50	81.82	82.69	82.98	86.27	79.17	0.00%	66.67	81.25	79.03	82.14
2017年	75.47	80.95	89.47	50.00	70.59	86.76	69.70	67.65	78.57	80.49	64.91	81.58	93.75	86.36	81.61	81.58	78.95	72.55	50.00	62.50	76.34	60.00	75.00	71.43	74.34	88.46	50.00	73.17	79.17	81.65	74.19
2018年	61.82	73.71	71.79	62.50	57.08	67.57	53.85	72.97	76.24	75.11	66.67	73.17	60.87	73.17	70.21	51.16	68.75	57.38	71.43	77.78	71.64	73.68	69.09	66.13	59.68	70.00	0.00%	55.81	62.00	75.00	65.63

Chapter Three

Quality Assurance

In order to implement the healthy China strategy and the national decisions on blood management, health authorities at all levels prioritized blood safety. Guided by the principles of "random selection of inspectors and the inspected" and "public disclosure of the results," the National Health Commission carried out the 2018 technical verification of blood safety at establishments with long-term mechanisms for government-led voluntary blood donation, the clinical use of blood and quality management. Meanwhile, with an emphasis on strengthening blood nucleic acid detection and quality management across the entire process of blood collection and supply, all localities advanced blood management, promoted IT applications, and innovated working modes to ensure blood safety.

I. Progress in the Technical Verification of Blood Safety

On the one hand, the National Health Commission continued to improve the technical procedures, standards and specifications of blood centers. It also gave instructions to local governments to promote personnel training and assessment, advance the information system of blood management, and strengthen the screening system for high-risk blood donors. On the other hand, according to the requirements of "reforms to streamline the administration, relegate power, improve regulation and upgrade services" and to bolster the awareness of blood safety and responsibility, the National Health Commission carried out the technical verification of blood safety involving 10 provinces (as well as autonomous regions and municipalities directly under the central government) in 2018, which covered the laws and regulations on blood safety, quality management specifications and technical operation procedures. It also engaged in on-site inspections and in-depth exchanges with blood centers, plasma centers and medical institutions. During the quality management meeting for nationwide plasma centers held in Kunming, the spirit of the meeting was announced, the problems found during the technical verification of blood safety were reported and their solutions were proposed.

II. Rigorous Law Enforcement and Supervision of Blood Safety at All Levels

With the focus on improving blood safety and the ability to guarantee the blood supply, all provinces (as well as autonomous regions and municipalities directly under the central government) carried out annual verification to review the daily operation of blood centers and plasma centers, especially during the certificate renewal period. In this way, operations under the relevant laws and regulations were strengthened. Meanwhile, the department of comprehensive law-enforcement and health supervision at the provincial, municipal and county levels inspected the blood centers, hospitals and plasma centers on both regular and irregular bases. The inspections were conducted once, twice and fourth times at three levels respectively. The combination of daily supervision and special inspections was guaranteed. All these efforts helped promote the lawful and regulated operation system and improved the evaluation system for blood collection and supply institutions. In addition, strict inspections were ensured across key aspects regarding blood safety so that hidden dangers could be found in time. Then, time limits for rectification were proposed regarding the reported results of supervision and inspection. All local authorities were encouraged to solve problems in various ways in a timely manner and to submit rectification reports. Through supervision and inspection, the quality of blood management was further improved to ensure the safety of clinical blood use.

III. The Continuous Optimization of Prevention and Control Measures for Blood Safety

First, all provinces (as well as autonomous regions and municipalities directly under the central government) conducted regular internal auditing and EQA to improve laboratory testing capacity. Second, the system for quality assessment and standards was constantly strengthened. Beijing applied for the formulation of the *Technical Standards for the Clinical Use of Blood at Beijing Healthcare Institutions*, and it revised quality management documents such as the *Implementation Rules of Inspections for the Blood Transfusion Departments at Beijing Healthcare Institutions* and *Quality Assessment Indicators for Blood Transfusion Departments or Blood Banks in Beijing Healthcare Institutions*. Third, IT applications were further enhanced. Jiangsu set up a provincial platform for blood administrative information management, an online fee reductions and exemptions platform for blood use in different localities, and provincial management platforms for donor quarantine and blood redistribution. In addition, Gansu established a warning information platform for blood use. Fourth, training regarding each link of blood collection and supply was thoroughly developed through a variety of training courses with ample content. Fifth, sampling inspections of blood quality were intensified. The blood (plasma) collected by blood collection and supply institutions in Anhui and Guangxi was regularly sampled and then monitored for four viruses, including hepatitis B, hepatitis C, HIV and syphilis . Sixth, the management system for bad records was advanced. Guangxi and Sichuan respectively introduced the *Scoring System for Bad Records of Blood Quality Assessment at Blood Collection and Supply Institutions in Guangxi*, the *Management Measures on the Scoring System for Bad Operations at Plasma Centers in Sichuan Province* and the *Management Measures on the Scoring System for Bad Operations at Healthcare Institutions in Sichuan Province*. The scoring of bad records was taken as a demerit during technical review. In this way, blood collection and supply institutions were urged to improve their daily operations and management.

2018 年国家血液安全报告

China's Report on Blood Safety 2018

Section Six

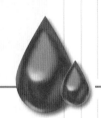

Blood Supply and Blood for Clinical Use

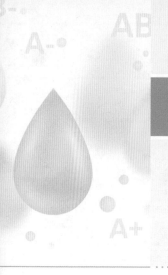

Chapter One

Blood Components Supply

Blood component transfusion is one of the important indexes to measure the technical advancement of blood transfusion in a country, a region or a hospital. Since the promulgation of the *Law of Blood Donation* in 1998, blood transfusion medicine has been developing steadily, with the proportion of blood component transfusion increasing year by year. In 2018, the separation rate of blood components in China's blood establishments reached 99.82%.

I. The Total Supply of Blood Components Increased Year by Year

At present, China's blood supply for clinical use mainly includes the following types: whole blood, erythrocyte components, platelet components and plasma components.

Whole blood: In 2018, 42,000 units of whole blood were issued from blood centers in China, an increase of 36.1% over 2017 (Figure 6-1).

Erythrocyte components. These mainly include erythrocyte in additive solution, washed erythrocyte, thawed erythrocyte, leukocytes reduced erythrocyte and irradiated erythrocyte. In 2018, 22.607 million units of erythrocyte components were supplied by blood centers in China, an increase of 2.8% over 2017. Leukocytes reduced erythrocyte accounted for the largest proportion (66.2%) of all erythrocyte components issued from blood centers in China, followed by erythrocyte in additive solution (29.2%) (Figure 6-2).

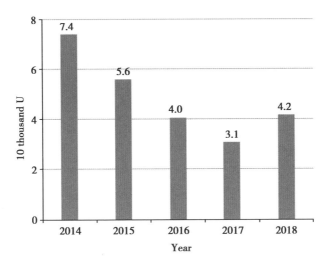

Figure 6-1   The volume of clinical whole blood supply, 2014-2018

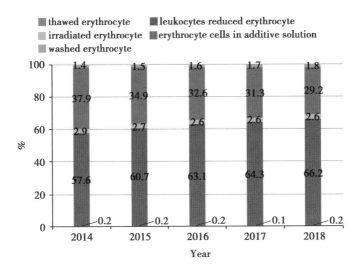

Figure 6-2   Ratio of the clinical supply of erythrocyte
components by category, 2014-2018

Platelet components. These include apheresis platelets and platelet concentrate. From 2014 to 2018, the apheresis platelet supply was abundant and increased year by year. In 2018, 1.779 million units of apheresis platelets were collected from blood establishments in China, a growth of 10.2% over 2017. The supply of platelet concentrate was small. In 2018,

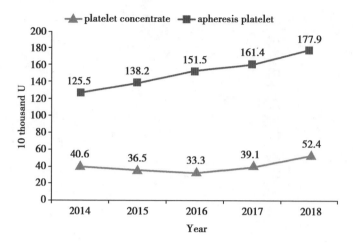

Figure 6-3   The number of clinical apheresis platelets and
platelet concentrate supply, 2014-2018

524,000 units of platelet concentrate were collected from blood centers in
China, up 34.1% over 2017 (Figure 6-3).

Plasma components. These mainly include fresh frozen plasma,
frozen plasma and virally inactive plasma. In 2018, 21.322 million units of
plasma components were issued from blood centers in China, an increase
of 12.4% over 2017 (Figure 6-4).

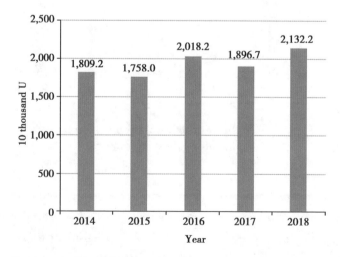

Figure 6-4   The volume of clinical plasma supply, 2014-2018

The utilization rate of formed elements is one of the important indexes to evaluate the overall utilization and quality management of blood at blood centers. Since 2016, China has seen an increase in the utilization rate of formed elements. The utilization rate in 2018 was 102.13%, 0.5 percentage points higher than that of 2017 (Figure 6-5).

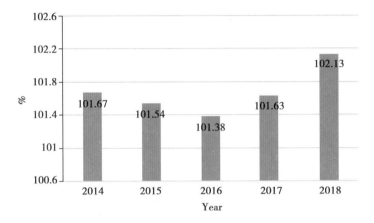

Figure 6-5   The utilization rate of formed elements, 2014-2018

II. Balance in Blood Supply and Collection Promoted by Redistribution

In 2018, various regions in China further promoted balance in blood supply and collection by redistribution, enhancing blood security and strengthening inventory management (Figure 6-6).

In recent years, the incidence of blood redistribution among different areas of China increased year by year and mainly took place within one province (Figure 6-7).

III. Blood Inventory Management Improved

Discarded blood is divided into two cases: test-based discarding and physical discarding. Test-based discarded blood refers to unqualified blood from laboratory testing and CUE, whereas physical discarded blood refers to rejected blood products due to abnormal appearance (chylaemia, blood bag damage, etc.) and otherwise qualified blood products rejected for being past their shelf life. Physical discarded blood is one of the indexes for assessing the management of blood establishments.

In 2018, the volume of physical discarded blood was 1.512 million

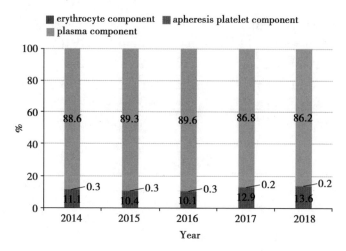

Figure 6-6   Ratio of blood stock by category, 2014-2018

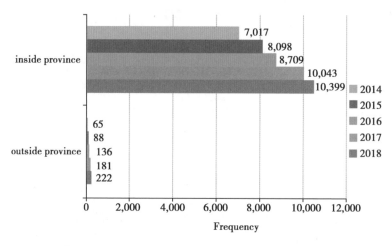

Figure 6-7   Frequency of blood transfers, 2014-2018

units, 1.2% less than the volume of physical discarded blood in 2017. In addition, the rate of physical discarded blood was 3.1%, a decrease of 0.3 percentage points over that of 2017 (Figure 6-8).

In 2018, physical discarded blood, mainly caused by abnormal appearances, accounted for 96.5% of all discarded blood, a growth of 0.4 percentage points over that of 2017 (Figure 6-9).

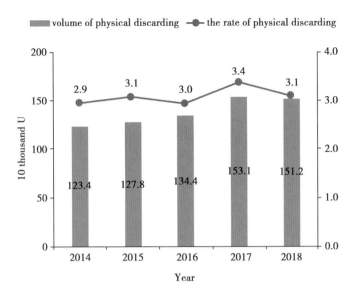

Figure 6-8   Physical discarded blood, 2014-2018

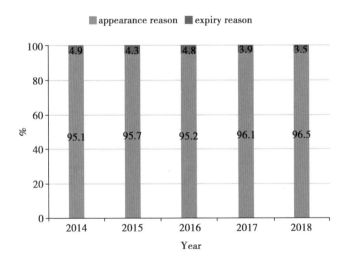

Figure 6-9   Ratio of physical discarded blood by reason, 2014-2018

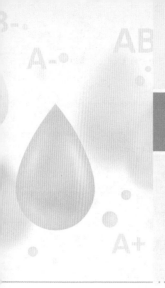

Chapter Two

Blood for Clinical Use

According to the 2018 statistical bulletin on the development of health care services in China, in 2018, the total number of patients received and inpatients at health care institutions grew by 130 million and 10.17 million, respectively, over the prior year. With improved medical services, the national per capita blood consumption was 3.3ml, 0.1ml higher than that of 2017; platelet consumption per ten thousand people was 13.1 units, an increase of 1.2 units compared with 11.9 units in 2017. The administrative department of health care focused on enhancing law-based governance, blood supply, blood safety and the rational use of blood, and it made multi-step and multi-action plans to keep the management of blood for clinical use up to date with the times and adapted to the development needs of the new era.

I. Continuous Improvement in Managing Blood for Clinical Use

(I) Constant Upgrade of the Systems and Regulations of Managing Blood for Clinical Use

Notice on Printing and Distributing the Key Points of the Core System of Medical Quality and Safety (by MOH No. 8 [2018]) issued by the National Health Commission of the PRC, highlighted the audit system of blood for clinical use as one of the 18 core systems of medical quality and safety. While emphasizing the importance of the management of blood for clinical use, it also standardized the definition, content, requirements, operating procedures and implementation effects of the core system of medical institutions on the national level. The promulgation of *Transfusion of Whole Blood and Blood Components* (WS/T 623—2108) in 2018 marked Chinese entrance on the stage of standardization for blood in clinical use, further regulating the clinical use of blood. Based on the *Management Measures on the Clinical Use of Blood* by Healthcare Institutions and the *Technical Standards for Clinical Blood Transfusion* and other documents, the provincial health administrative departments in Nei Mongol, Hebei, Henan, Hubei, Shaanxi, Chongqing, Liaoning, Qinghai, Xinjiang, Hainan and other provinces formulated or revised their management methods, clinical transfusion guidelines, quality safety manuals, quality evaluation standards, management guidelines and audit criteria of blood for clinical use at medical institutions in their respective administrative regions, effectively regulating the management of blood for clinical use within their jurisdiction.

(II) Increasingly Strict Admission of Blood for Clinical Use in Medical Institutions

Beijing, Jilin, Ningxia, Guizhou and other provinces (as well as autonomous regions and municipalities directly under the central government) strengthened the standardized and responsible management of blood for clinical use in medical institutions by strictly managing the admission of new medical institutions that apply for clinical blood use or new blood transfusion departments (blood banks) of medical institutions, as well as by verifying or signing agreements with medical institutions that are qualified.

(III) Continual Enhancement of Medical Staff Awareness of Rational Blood Use

Anhui, Guangxi, Hunan and other provinces (and autonomous regions) as well as the Xinjiang Production and Construction Corps, supervised the medical institutions within their jurisdictions by displaying or revealing the blood use of medical institutions and other management methods, strengthening the management of blood for clinical use and the awareness of medical staff, and thus saving blood.

II. Constant Boost in the Quality Control of Blood for Clinical Use

Provincial centers for the quality control of blood for clinical use assisted the health administrative department to continuously strengthen the capability building of blood for clinical use in medical institutions by actively carrying out different tasks. By the end of 2018, 30 provincial administrative units in China had set up provincial quality control centers for blood for clinical use, among which 2 provincial quality control centers for blood for clinical use in Tianjin and the Xinjiang Production and Construction Corps achieved excellence in an assessment by the National Health Commission. Through the continuous promotion of the concept and experience of the rational use of clinical blood, provinces (as well as autonomous regions and municipalities directly under the central government) effectively reduced the occurrence of intraoperative bleeding and adverse reactions during blood transfusion, ensuring the blood use safety of patients.

(I) The Steady Upgrade of the Quality Control System for Clinical Blood Transfusion

By the end of 2018, except for Jiangxi province and the Xizang Zizhiqu, which have not yet established provincial quality control centers for blood for clinical use, other provincial quality control centers for blood for clinical use have improved the building of provincial and municipal quality control centers for blood for clinical use under the leadership of the health administrative department of provinces (as well as autonomous regions and municipalities directly under the central government). Among them, Fujian province has completed the construction of quality control centers in 9 cities; Sichuan province has gradually developed a third-tier quality control network for blood for clinical use in the province, and it has set up 151 county/district level quality control centers for blood for clinical use as of July 2018.

(II) The Constant Enhancement of the Regular Supervision of Blood for Clinical Use

Provincial quality control centers for blood for clinical use carried out, both regularly and irregularly, means of technical verification of blood safety, as well as the supervision, inspection and investigation of blood for clinical use in medical institutions, guiding medical institutions within their jurisdiction on the rational and safe use of blood.

(III) The Gradual Strengthening of the Human Resources for Blood Transfusion at Medical Institutions

Provincial quality control centers for blood for clinical use strengthened human resources for blood transfusion at medical institutions within their jurisdictions through training and the exchange of policies, theories and technical expertise, as well as by sharing high-quality resources with community stakeholders.

III. The Continuous Promotion of New Technologies and Methods for Blood for Clinical Use

Provincial health administrative departments guided and promoted clinical departments to perform well-developed and reliable, minimally invasive surgeries that lead to small wounds and less bleeding, so as to achieve minimized blood use for surgery and targeted and cost-effective clinical blood use, reducing the blood demand for surgery and intraoperative bleeding. The promotion of retrieved and stored autologous blood transfusion, blood replacement therapy, patient blood management (PBM) and other blood protection methods not only improved the safety of blood for clinical use, but also effectively saved blood.

According to the data on the technical verification of blood safety by the National Health Commission of the PRC in 2018 (of which the data for Xizang Zizhiqu and Hainan were excluded), through the continuous promotion of new technologies of blood protection and new methods of blood management, tertiary hospitals that were verified and investigated in all provinces (as well as autonomous regions and municipalities directly under the central government)saw the increasing number of discharged patients and operations on inpatients (Figure 6-10), little changing in the amount of almost all blood components used except for a rising plasma consumption (Figure 6-11).

In eastern China (including Beijing, Tianjin, Hebei, Liaoning, Shanghai, Jiangsu, Zhejiang, Fujian, Shandong, Guangdong and Hainan, as below), the amount of erythrocyte and plasma used at the investigated tertiary hospitals remained almost unchanged, platelets consumption increased slightly, and cryoprecipitate consumption decreased. In the central region (including Shanxi, Jilin, Heilongjiang, Anhui, Jiangxi, Henan, Hubei, Hunan, as below), erythrocyte dosages were almost the same, with

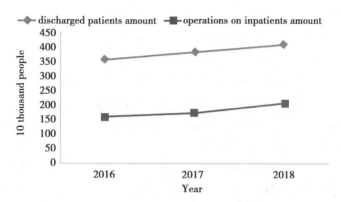

Figure 6-10   Total amount of discharged patients and
operations on inpatients at the tertiary hospitals investigated
in the 2018 technical verification of blood safety, 2016-2018

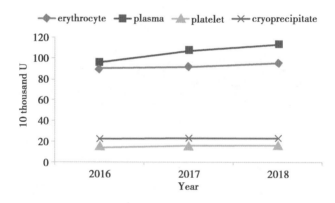

Figure 6-11   Total amount of blood components used at the
investigated tertiary hospitals in the 2018 technical verification
of blood safety, 2016-2018

slight growth in the other blood components. In western China (including
Sichuan, Chongqing, Guizhou, Yunnan, Xizang, Shaanxi, Gansu, Qinghai,
Ningxia, Xinjiang, Guangxi, Nei Mongol, as below), except for a small rise
in the amount of plasma consumption, other blood components remained
stable (Figure 6-12 to Figure 6-15).

Various technologies adopted by medical institutions can reduce
unnecessary blood preparation and transfusion, as well as the risks related
to using blood for clinical use. For example, the Cancer Hospital of the
Chinese Academy of Medical Sciences (hereinafter referred to as the

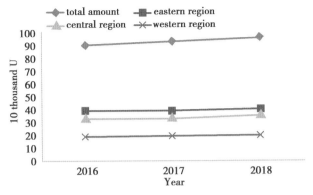

Figure 6-12   Total amount of erythrocyte used at the investigated tertiary hospitals in different regions in the 2018 technical verification of blood safety, 2016-2018

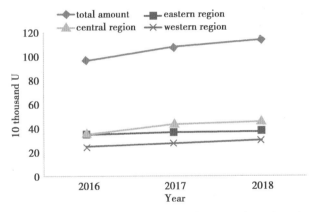

Figure 6-13   Total amount of plasma used at the investigated tertiary hospitals in different regions in the 2018 technical verification of blood safety, 2016-2018

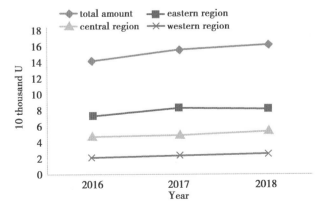

Figure 6-14   Total amount of platelets used at the investigated tertiary hospitals in different regions in the 2018 technical verification of blood safety, 2016-2018

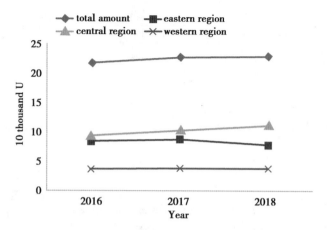

Figure 6-15   Total amount of cryoprecipitate used at the
investigated tertiary hospitals in different regions in the 2018
technical verification of blood safety, 2016-2018

Cancer Hospital) has used preoperative arterial embolization on tumors
with abundant blood supply, temporary balloon occlusion, interventional
embolization on hemorrhaging tumors and other interventional therapies.
Preoperative arterial embolization and temporary balloon occlusion can
significantly reduce bleeding in operations on tumors with abundant blood
supply. The wide application of this technology to surgical departments
for tumor treatment can lower unnecessary blood preparation and
transfusion. For patients with acute hemorrhaging, angiography can
locate the bleeding. In addition, interventional embolization of tumor
hemorrhaging results in smaller wounds and better hemostasis effects.
In 2018, more than 200 cases of tumor hemorrhaging were treated by
interventional embolization in the interventional therapy department of
the Cancer Hospital. The technique's great hemostasis effect significantly
reduced clinical blood consumption.

IV. Constant Enhancement of the Standardization of Blood for Clinical Use

With the promotion of health administrative departments of different
regions and provincial quality control centers for blood for clinical use,
the clinical blood use in medical institutions has improved year by year.
According to the technical verification data on blood safety by the National

Health Commission of the PRC in 2018, with the increasing number of discharged patients and operations on inpatients, the total amount of per operation blood consumption, the per capita blood consumption of discharged patients, the percentage of blood transfusion patients, the per capita blood consumption of blood transfusion patients and the per operation table platelet consumption over the three years from 2016 to 2018 all showed a downward trend at the investigated tertiary hospitals. The clinical rational use of blood at the investigated hospitals was boosted (Figure 6-16 to Figure 6-20).

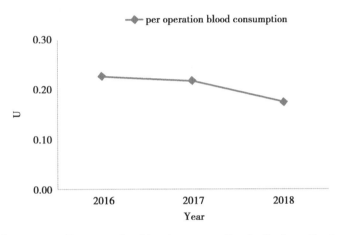

Figure 6-16 Per operation blood consumption in the investigated hospitals in the 2018 technical verification of blood safety, 2016-2018

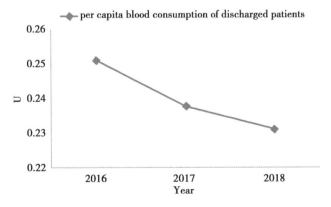

Figure 6-17 Per capita blood consumption of discharged patients in the investigated hospitals of the 2018 technical verification of blood safety, 2016-2018

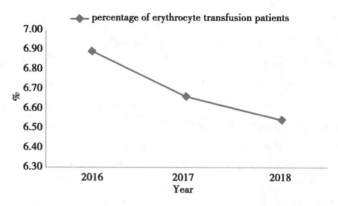

Figure 6-18   Percentage of blood transfusion patients in the investigated
hospitals in the 2018 technical verification of blood safety, 2016-2018

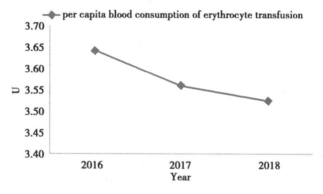

Figure 6-19   Per capita blood consumption of erythrocyte transfusion
patients in the investigated hospitals of the 2018 technical verification of
blood safety, 2016-2018

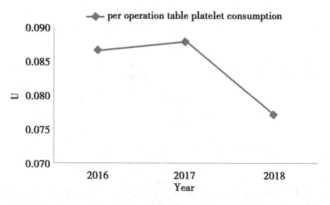

Figure 6-20   Per operation table platelet consumption in the investigated
hospitals of the 2018 technical verification of blood safety, 2016-2018

Regionally, the investigated tertiary hospitals in the eastern central and western regions all saw a downward trend in per operation blood consumption and per capita blood consumption of discharged patients (Figure 6-21 and Figure 6-22). The percentage of blood transfusion patients increased in the western region, slightly decreased in the central region and significantly dropped in the eastern region (Figure 6-23). The per capita blood consumption of blood transfusion patients declined in the western region and remained unstable in the central and

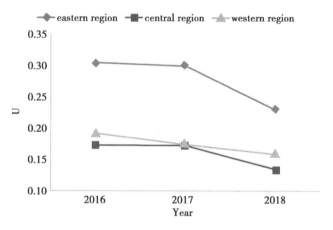

Figure 6-21   Per operation blood consumption in the investigated hospitals over past three years in different regions in the 2018 technical verification of blood safety

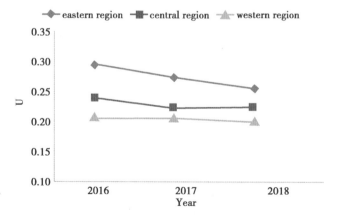

Figure 6-22   Per capita blood consumption of discharged patients in the investigated hospitals over past three years in different regions of the 2018 technical verification of blood safety

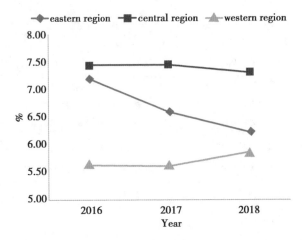

Figure 6-23   Percentage of blood transfusion patients in the investigated hospitals over past three years in different regions in the 2018 technical verification of blood safety

eastern regions(Figure 6-24). The per operation table platelet consumption fell off overall, with a relatively sharp decline in the eastern region in 2018 followed by slight growth in 2017, a slow falling trend in the central region, and little change in the western region over almost three years (Figure 6-25).

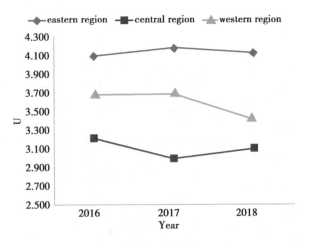

Figure 6-24   Per capita blood consumption of blood transfusion patients in the investigated hospitals over past three years in different regions of the 2018 technical verification of blood safety

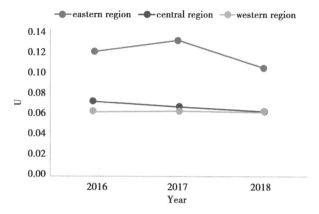

Figure 6-25   Per operating table platelet consumption in
the investigated hospitals over past three years in different
regions in the 2018 technical verification of blood safety

2018 年国家血液安全报告

China's Report on Blood Safety 2018

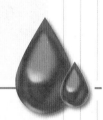

Plasmapheresis
Centers

I. There was a continuous increase in plasmapheresis centers

In 2018, 25 provinces, autonomous regions or municipalities directly under the central government in China set up plasmapheresis centers. Among them, in 2018 Liaoning province, Yunnan province and Fujian province approved the establishment of plasmapheresis centers for the first time and began the practice. In Sichuan, Guangdong, Guangxi and other provinces or autonomous regions, the number of plasmapheresis centers exceeded 20 (Figure 7-1).

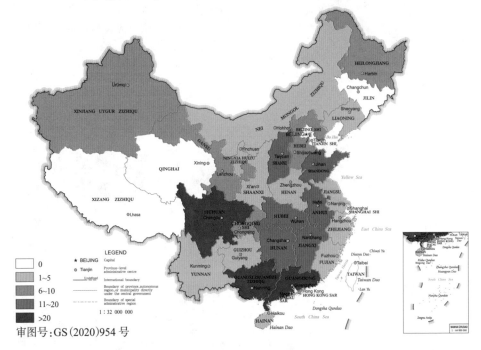

审图号:GS (2020)954 号

Figure 7-1   Distribution of plasmapheresis centers in 2018
(Remark: the data of this figure do not include HONG KONG SAR, MACAU SAR and TAIWAN Province.)

II. There was a steady increase in raw plasma collection

In 2018, China collected 8,343 tons of raw plasma, an increase of 8.1% respectively, compared with the prior year (Figure 7-2). There were 5 plasmapheresis centers that had an annual volume of over 100 tons.

The largest source of raw plasma in China was Sichuan province, followed by Guangxi Zhuangzu Zizhiqu and Shandong provinces (Figure 7-3).

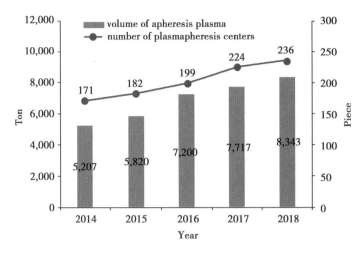

Figure 7-2   Volume of apheresis plasma and the number of
plasmapheresis centers, 2014—2018

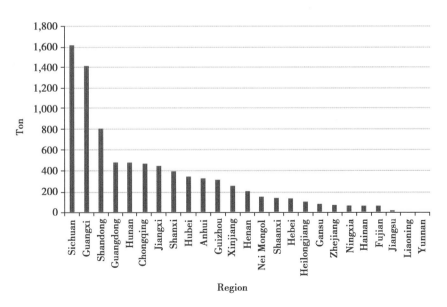

Figure 7-3   Volume of apheresis plasma by region in 2018

2018 年国家血液安全报告

China's Report on Blood Safety 2018

Section Eight

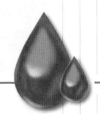

Transfusion
Medicine:
Research and
Education

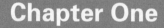

Chapter One

Transfusion Medicine:
Research and Education

I. Scientific and Technological Innovation Pushed the Industry Forward

In 2018, 13 national level blood industry related scientific research projects (including support from the National Natural Science Foundation) were approved with a total of 16.29 million yuan in funds, according to a survey and statistics of 24 provincial blood centers, 166 municipal blood centers, 3 medical institutions and 2 scientific research institutions. The projects were mainly initiated by the Blood Transfusion Research Institute of the Chinese Academy of Medical Sciences and the Health Service and Blood Research Center of the Military Medical Research Institute. The main research fields were on blood cells and transfusion-transmitted diseases. 27 provincial and ministerial level scientific research projects with a total funding of about 2.3 million yuan were also approved. The approved projects were mostly from the Blood Transfusion Research Institute of the Chinese Academy of Medical Sciences, the Health Service and Blood Research Center of the Military Medical Research Institute and the PLA General Hospital, etc, The research focused on blood cells, transfusion-transmitted diseases, clinical transfusion and information management (Figure 8-1).

II. Steady Growth of Scientific and Technological Achievements

A total of 9 provincial and ministerial scientific and technological awards were granted to the institutions in the blood transfusion industry (Figure 8-2)

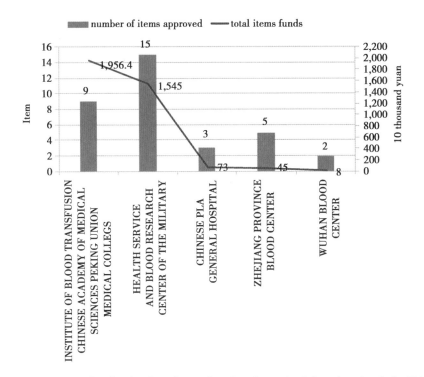

Figure 8-1   Top five institutions by national and provincial project funds in 2018

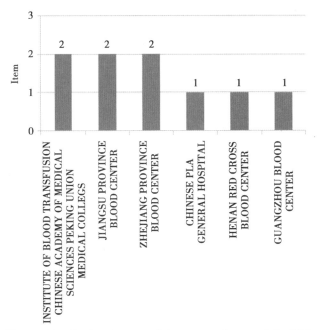

Figure 8-2   Institutions receiving research awards in 2018

for projects including research on new technology and screening strategies for blood borne pathogens prevention and control, the mechanism of adverse reactions during blood transfusion, etc. 23 national invention patents and 15 patents on utility models (Figure 8-3) were approved and authorized, mainly in the fields of blood transport devices, testing reagents and methods.

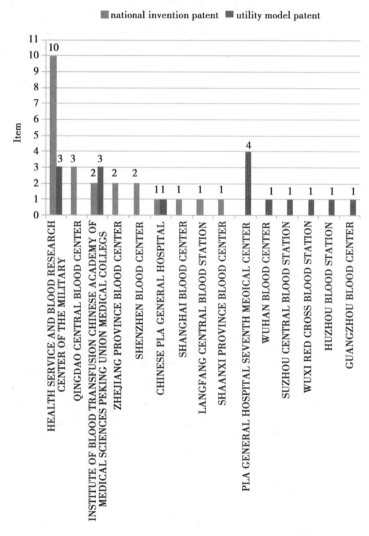

Figure 8-3   Institutions obtaining patents in 2018

III. The Quality of Research Papers Improved

According to incomplete statistics, in 2018 there were 127 SCI research papers published by Chinese researchers of transfusion medicine as the first author or corresponding author, with an impact factor reaching 388 points. Among those papers, the majority were published by researchers of the Institute of Blood Transfusion of the Chinese Academy of Medical Sciences (IBT/CAMS) (27 papers, Figure 8-4). The article in *Hepatology* had the single highest impact factor (IF 14.079). The published papers covered the areas of blood immunology, epidemiology, clinical blood transfusion, materials chemistry, biochemistry and molecular biology, as well as other topics in blood transfusion medicine. These SCI papers were published in about 50 English-language journals (or magazines), including *HLA*, *Transfusion* and other high-impact professional journals in the blood transfusion medicine industry (Figure 8-5). 367 and 325 articles were published in core Chinese and non-Chinese journals, respectively.

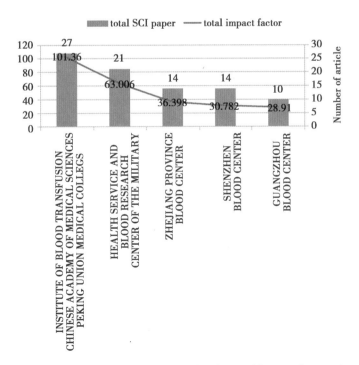

Figure 8-4   Top five institutions by the total impact factor of
SCI article publications in 2018

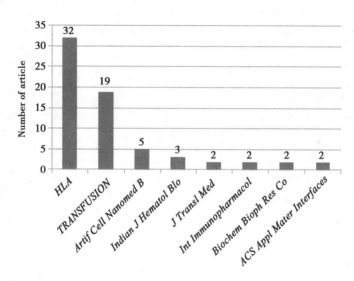

Figure 8-5   Top eight SCI journals by the number of articles published in 2018

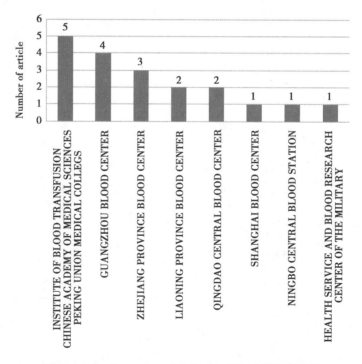

Figure 8-6   Journals published in *TRANSFUSION*

IV. The Influence of Specialized Publications Continued to Grow

In 2018, a total of more than 10 monographs were published, including *China's Report on Blood Safety 2017*, the *Legalization Process of Blood Management, Clinical Blood Transfusion Technical Manual, Blood Establishments Sterilization and Contamination Management, and Blood Composition Preparation, and Use and Quality Assurance Guide. China's Report on Blood Safety 2017*, written and edited by experts and professionals of the National Health Commission of the PRC once again, as a continuation of the 2016 report, elaborated on the overall situation of blood collection and supply in China in 2017. To celebrate the 20th anniversary of the promulgation and implementation of the *Law of Blood Donation*, the *Legalization Process of Blood Management* was jointly written by experts from the Chinese Academy of Medical Sciences and the National Health Commission. This work reflected upon the legalization process of blood management, summarized the achievements of blood safety work since the implementation of the *Law of Blood Donation* in China, analyzed the challenges in the new era, and referred to the methods and approaches of blood management by foreign counterparts. The work also analyzed ideas and suggestions for the legal development of blood management in China and presented the Chinese model and experience of blood management, all of which provided new theories and methods for the next step of blood management in China.

Chapter Two

Transfusion Medicine Education

In 2018, a total of 20,000 trainees attended more than 130 provincial- and national-level continuing education training courses. Among them, the number of national continuing education training courses declined, while the number of provincial-level courses increased significantly. In addition, the resources for continuing education became more accessible. These training courses witnessed the participation of blood services institutions, medical institutions and research institutions at all levels. Courses covered management, recruitment, testing and quality control, and they provided a

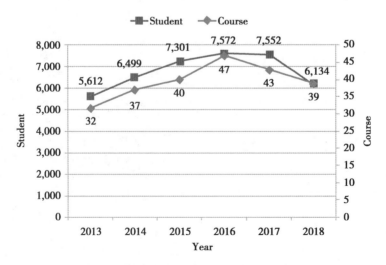

Figure 8-7　National continuing education courses

multitude of learning and training opportunities for grassroots transfusion practitioners. Continuing education and training greatly improved the overall service level of the industry(Figure 8-7 to Figure 8-9).

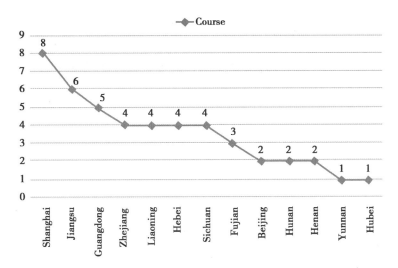

Figure 8-8   Regional distribution of national continuing education courses in 2018

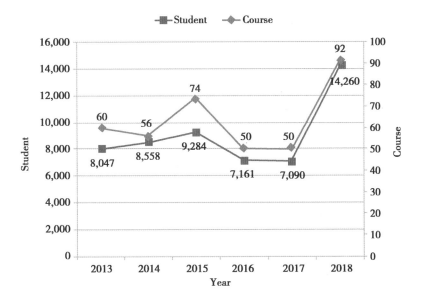

Figure 8-9   Provincial continuing education courses

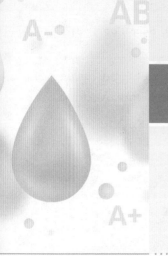

Chapter Three

Academic Exchange and International Cooperation

In 2018, more than 50 national exchange programs were carried out with more than 8,000 participants. One international academic event was attended by about thirty international participants. In addition, more than 20 participants gave speeches at international academic conferences, sharing the Chinese experience in the field of transfusion medicine.

I. Increased International Influence

From December 11 to 14, 2017, the Fourth APEC Blood Safety Policy Forum and Quality Workshop was held in Jakarta, Indonesia. The Ministry of Health of Indonesia and the Asia Pacific Economic Cooperation (APEC) Life Sciences Innovation Forum (LSIF) Blood Safety Network co-hosted the event. Relevant principals and industry experts from the Bureau of Medical Administration of the National Health Commission were invited to participate in the event. They introduced China's model and experience in blood supply and safety to the economies of the Asia Pacific region, which was well received by most of the participating countries. At the same time, the achievements and challenges in non-remunerated blood donation and blood safety, especially the experience in policy making and its implementation, were also presented, followed by an elaborate exchange of views and a discussion of blood quality management.

From May 16 to 18, 2018, the World Health Organization Cooperation

Center and Key Implementing Partners Meeting on Blood and Transfusion Safety jointly organized by the Service Delivery and Safety (SDS) of the WHO and the Shanghai Blood Center/WHO Blood Transfusion Cooperation Center was held in Shanghai. 27 heads and officials of WHO headquarters, WHO regional offices, national representative offices, trade associations and international organizations in the field of blood transfusion attended the meeting. The aim of the meeting was to coordinate WHO Cooperation Centers and key implementing partners' efforts in supporting WHO blood safety and supply security at the global, regional and national levels. The meeting reviewed the global context and the successful experience in the policies and strategies for the building of blood safety systems, the efforts made by countries in promoting the "Melbourne Declaration-100% non-remunerated blood donation" , how to obtain more secure and safe blood supplies, and the reasonable and fair use of blood. At the same time, cooperation between Chinese and foreign governments was further explored , as well as research institutes, in terms of blood and transfusion safety in addition to the chances brought about by the "Belt and Road initiative."

From June 12 to 13, 2018, the Plasma Protein 2018 Summit (PPF2018) was held in Washington D.C., the United States. The meeting was hosted by the Plasma Protein Therapeutics Association (PPTA). A total of 260 government officials, research experts, representatives from blood centers, plasma centers, blood product enterprises and related associations, as well as doctors and patient representatives from the United States, Canada, the United Kingdom, Germany, India, Republic of Korea and China, attended the summit. Relevant officials and industry experts of the Bureau of Medical Administration of the National Health Commission were invited to attend the meeting.

From July 10 to 12, 2018, the International Blood Early Warning Conference was held in Manchester, the United Kingdom. The Adverse Reaction Mechanism of the Blood Transfusion Research Group funded by the Medicine, Health and Innovation Program of the Chinese Academy of Medical Sciences was invited to attend the meeting. At the meeting, progress made in the research on adverse reactions during blood transfusion and blood safety management in China was introduced, in addition to the progress made towards blood safety early warning.

II. Continuous Expansion of International Modes of Cooperation

In 2018, some of China's blood collection and supply institutions and medical institutions also carried out international exchanges and cooperation, with deepening fields of cooperation and innovative cooperation modes. Among these exchanges, Liaoning Provincial Blood Center and the National Institute of Blood Transfusion (INTS) of France carried out research cooperation on the molecular properties, pathogenesis and infectivity of OBI. Shanghai Blood Center and Mongolia National Medical Center of Blood Transfusion jointly signed a "Training Course Agreement on Immunohematology Tests and Related Tests of Cord Blood Bank and Hematopoietic Stem Cell Bank" to provide relevant skills training for personnel at Mongolia National Medical Center of Blood Transfusion. Chengdu Municipal Blood Center and Stanford Blood Center signed a cooperation framework agreement. The agreement stipulates that the two sides will carry out extensive and in-depth cooperative research in the fields of blood donor recruitment, blood quality management, the prevention of blood-borne diseases, HLA detection, platelet antigen typing, red cell immune serology, etc, and the two will work together to improve blood safety and blood applications. Yunnan Kunming Municipal Blood Center signed a framework agreement on scientific research cooperation with Laos National Red Cross Society and National Blood Transfusion Center.

In 2018, China's blood collection and supply institutions sent a total number of 50 staff to visit the United States, Japan, Canada, Australia and Israel for learning and medium- and long-term training in transfusion medicine, experimental technology and blood management. At the same time, 59 experts from the National Blood Center of Canada, Stanford University, the National Blood Transfusion Research Institute of France, the National Serology Reference Laboratory of Australia and other institutions came to China for exchange, visit, training and lecture.

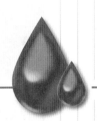

The Continuous Development of Blood Collection and Supply in Xizang Zizhiqu

In recent years, under the great attention and support of the Communist Party of China and the State, and with donor match-making at its core, blood collection and supply in the Xizang Zizhiqu made remarkable progress. A supportive environment for participation in voluntary non-remunerated blood donation underwent daily improvement, the number and scope of blood collection and supply institutions across the entire region expanded, and the total blood supply and the proportion of component blood supply grew significantly. Xizang Zizhiqu implemented independent blood nucleic acid testing, and the capacity for blood safety protection was continuously improved.

I. Initial Progress of Group Assistance to Xizang Zizhiqu

Since the former Ministry of Health held the "Coordination Conference for Tailored Assistance and Signing Ceremony of Assistance for Xizang Zizhiqu's Blood Collection and Supply" in Lhasa in 2011, as well as, in particular, the conference on "group" tailored assistance to Xizang Zizhiqu's blood collection and supply in 2015, governments at all levels attached increasing importance to the region's blood collection and supply industry. Under the unified deployment of the National Health Commission of the PRC, it was determined that from July 2017, 8 provinces and municipalities, namely Jiangsu, Anhui, Shaanxi, Guangdong, Sichuan, Beijing, Shanghai and Chongqing would provide tailored assistance to Xizang Zizhiqu, in order to comprehensively promote blood collection and supply services in Xizang Zizhiqu.

II. Greater Importance Attached by the Government of the Xizang Zizhiqu

The Health Commission of Xizang Zizhiqu played an active part in this course of events. On the one hand, it increased investment in blood collection and supply infrastructure, allocating 9.3 million yuan to rebuild and expand the Blood Center of the Xizang Zizhiqu, as well as 6 million yuan to upgrade laboratories and other hardware equipment. On the other hand, it improved systemic standardization, and it revised and promulgated the Measures for Implementing the *Law of Blood Donation of the People's Republic of China in the Xizang Zizhiqu* which was implemented in January 2016.

III. Augmented Advocacy of Voluntary Non-remunerated Blood Donation

Under the support of the government of the Xizang Zizhiqu and the relevant departments, local blood collection and supply institutions held various publicity and advocacy events to continuously enhance and encourage the public's awareness and participation in voluntary non-remunerated blood donation. Every year, through mainstream media platforms such as radio, television, newspapers, magazines and modern communications services like QQ and WeChat, a diversity of events was launched to publicize voluntary non-remunerated blood donation on World Blood Donor Day, World Red Cross Day and other publicity days, as well as on festivals such as the Spring Festival and the New Year Day of Xizang Zizhiqu. The Measures for Implementing the *Law of Blood Donation of the People's Republic of China in the Xizang Zizhiqu*(both in Xizang Zizhiqu's language and Chinese) and the *Handbook for Voluntary Non-remunerated Blood Donation* and other popular science publicity materials were printed. In Xizang Zizhiqu Daily, Xizang Zizhiqu Business Daily, Lhasa Evening News and other newspapers, letters of thanks to voluntary non-remunerated blood donors were published. Voluntary non-remunerated blood donation videos were displayed on taxi LEDs, buses, cinemas and other large LED screens. Luo Zhen, a singer from an ensemble of the Xizang Zizhiqu, was selected as the image ambassador of Xizang Zizhiqu's voluntary non-remunerated blood donation by the Blood Center of the Xizang Zizhiqu. The short film, "Reshaping Life-Stories Behind Blood Donation in Xizang Zizhiqu," under the theme of voluntary non-remunerated blood donation, was created, and it won third place in the film category for excellent radio, film and television works of the National Health System.

IV. Full Coverage of Blood Collection and Supply Services

Before 2015, there were only 2 blood centers in the Xizang Zizhiqu; by 2018, the total blood centers in Xizang Zizhiqu numbered 7 (including those to be built), an increase of 2.5 times. 6 prefecture level cities and

1 region under the jurisdiction of the Xizang Zizhiqu concluded the establishment of blood collection and supply institutions, achieving the full coverage of blood collection and supply in the region (Table 9-1). Among them, Qamdo Regional Blood Bank (to be built) covered an area of 2,700m², about 1.4 times that of the Blood Center of the Xizang Zizhiqu. Since the implementation of tailored assistance, Xizang Zizhiqu has put a total of 8.55 million yuan of funds into use, and its infrastructure equipment is worth about 7.82 million yuan. By 2018, the total area of blood center housing in Xizang Zizhiqu had surpassed 7,000m², and major advances had been made in the planning and infrastructure of blood centers.

Table 9-1   Blood centers in the Xizang Zizhiqu

Name	Establishment time	Number of personnel	Staff	Actual on duty personnel	Floor area/m²
Xizang Zizhiqu Blood Center	2005	30	24	32	1,953
Nyingchi regional blood bank	2010	10	10	13	1,566
Ali regional blood bank	2015	10	6	9	—
Xigazê regional blood bank	2016	8	8	8	360
Nagqu regional blood bank	2017	12	11	11	723
Shannan regional blood bank	2017	10	10	10	—
Qamdo regional blood bank	To be built in 2018	9	9	17	2,700

V. Substantial Improvement of the Capacity to Guarantee a Safe Blood Supply

The volume of donation in new blood centers increased each year. With the development of blood collection, the number of whole blood donations and the amount of whole blood collection at Ali Regional Blood Bank, Nagqu Regional Blood Bank and Shannan Regional Blood Bank grew year by year. The annual growth rate of the total blood donations in 2015-2018 at Ali Regional Blood Bank reached 19.8%.

The total blood supply increased substantially. Xizang Zizhiqu established a mechanism focused on street donations, with group donations and other emergency donations as supplements, to guarantee its blood collection and supply. An emergency team of voluntary non-remunerated donors was set up, composed of public servants and staff from the health system, enterprises, institutions, schools and garrisoned troops. In addition, a team of blood donors with rare blood types was established to meet the demands of local healthcare services for the clinical use of blood. At the same time, the total clinical blood supply of the whole region went up significantly under the strong support of the national "group" assistance to Xizang Zizhiqu. From 2016 to 2018, Xizang Zizhiqu's cumulative blood transfers measured 32,293.5U (including suspended erythrocyte and plasma), accounting for 82% of the total clinical supply, which substantially eased local blood demand. In 2018, the total clinical supply of erythrocyte and plasma across the entire region reached 18,724 U (including blood for aid), an increase of 13,618.5U compared with 2014, registering an average annual growth rate of 38.38% (Figure 9-1). With its strengthening supply capacity, the scope of blood supply services across the entire region expanded. As of 2018, there were 71 blood supply medical

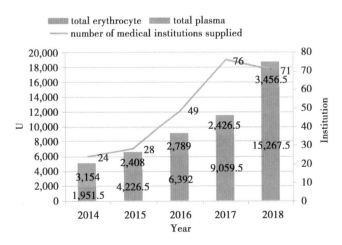

Figure 9-1   Total clinical blood supply in the Xizang Zizhiqu from 2014 to 2018

institutions in Xizang Zizhiqu, up 195.83% over 2014.

VI. The Remarkable Advancement of Blood Preparation Technology

Since the implementation of tailored assistance, there have been 38 batches and 400 instances of the study of blood management, enzyme immunoassays, component blood preparation, etc, in provinces and cities that have implemented tailored assistance. In addition, there have been more than 20 instances where provincial and municipal experts were stationed in Xizang Zizhiqu to train and teach local technical talent through 290 teacher-apprentice relationships, tremendously boosting the region's preparation and management of blood collection and supply. The total supply of clinical suspended erythrocyte across the entire region rose from 1,951.5U in 2014 to 15,267.5U in 2018 (including blood used for aid), an increase of 6.8 times. In 2013, the Blood Center of the Xizang Zizhiqu officially carried out the preparation of component blood, and the proportion of the component blood supply increased year by year (Figure 9-2); and by 2018, the clinical whole blood supply of the Blood Center of the Xizang Zizhiqu accounted for only 1.64% of the total.

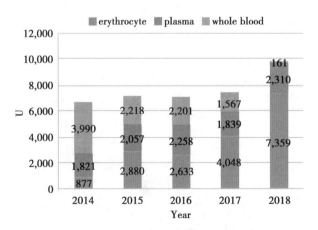

Figure 9-2   Component blood supply by the Blood Center of the Tibet Autonomous Region

VII. Constant Enhancement of Blood Safety

All blood establishments in Xizang Zizhiqu carried out enzyme immunoassays of blood-borne pathogens successively, effectively ensuring blood safety. Before the Blood Center of the Xizang Zizhiqu obtained qualifications for nucleic acid testing, the Chengdu Blood Center helped to launch centralized nucleic acid testing for 7,354 samples. The Blood Center of the Xizang Zizhiqu completed the upgrade of the nucleic acid testing laboratory and facilities in December 2016, and personnel training was completed in 2017. In January 2018, Xizang Zizhiqu obtained nucleic acid testing qualifications, and it launched testing in April of the same year, undertaking blood nucleic acid testing for the whole region (except the Ali Region). In April 2018, Nyingchi Regional Blood Bank started launching blood nucleic acid testing and result comparisons with the Blood Center of the Xizang Zizhiqu. By 2018, Xizang Zizhiqu had basically achieved full coverage of nucleic acid testing and effectively improved blood safety. At the same time, Xizang Zizhiqu strengthened the examination of the blood use qualifications of medical institutions. In 2018, during the blood use qualification examination for medical institutions, the qualifications of 10 medical institutions were cancelled in Shannan, further ensuring the safety of clinical blood use.

2018 年国家血液安全报告

China's Report on Blood Safety 2018

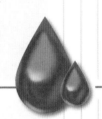

Conclusion and Future Prospects

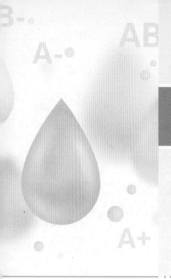

Chapter One

Main Achievements

In 2018, the total number of voluntary non-remunerated blood donors in China reached 14.79 million. The total volume of national blood donation was up to 25.06 million units. And the rate of blood donation reached 11.1 per thousand people. In 2018, the total number of voluntary non-remunerated blood donors and the volume of blood collection increased by 1.4% and 1.1% respectively compared with the prior year. China basically formed a working pattern of voluntary non-remunerated blood donation with complete system, scientific management, powerful guarantee as well as reasonable use, and achieved leapfrog development in various work.

I. The Blood Management Legal System was Gradually Improved and the Blood Safety Management Capacity Continued to Rise

The Law of Blood Donation was implemented all over the country, strengthening the leadership of organization and improving the working mechanism of voluntary non-remunerated blood donation. A three-level legal system of *The Law of Blood Donation* was gradually formed, consisting of national guidance, provincial regulations and municipal measures in response to that law. Health, finance, development and reform, publicity and other departments at all levels coordinated closely, aiming at promoting the regional voluntary non-remunerated blood donation with a strong sense of responsibility. With the continuous improvement of the legal system and scientific formulation of industry standards, blood safety has been effectively guaranteed.

II. The Social Environment of Voluntary Non-remunerated Blood Donation was Increasingly Active, and the Number of the Awardees for Voluntary Non-remunerated Blood Donation Increased Significantly

The publicity and recruitment of voluntary non-remunerated blood donors has been carried out all over the country, forming an encouraging social environment. On the Public Good Publicity Day of Voluntary Non-remunerated Blood Donation, a series of publicity activities for public good with various forms and rich contents were held from the state to all provinces (autonomous regions and municipalities directly under the central government), forming a positive public opinion atmosphere of voluntary non-remunerated blood donation. On December 12, 2018, National Health Commission of China, the Red Cross Society of China and the Health Bureau of the Logistics and Support Department of the Central Military Commission jointly issued The Decision on Awarding the Winners of Gold Medal and other Awards for 2016-2017 Voluntary Non-remunerated Blood Donation. In this year's commendation, the number of awardees for voluntary non-remunerated blood donation exceeded 390,000, an significant increase of 35.9% compared with the previous one. The continuous commendation activities and innovative incentive mechanisms for voluntary non-remunerated blood donors have made the work of voluntary non-remunerated blood donation widely understood and supported by the whole society. More and more people joined in the team of voluntary non-remunerated blood donors. The development of voluntary non-remunerated blood donation cause showed a healthy, sustainable and encouraging trend.

III. The Blood Collection and Supply Service Network Extended Continuously and the Blood Safety in Remote Areas was Improved

In order to guarantee the blood supply of our country, all localities reasonably allocated the construction of blood establishment according to the requirements of blood establishment's setup and planning. All localities continued to improve service facilities, enhance service awareness, optimize service processes, and revise the service system of blood establishment, focusing on blood donors and patients. By the end of 2018, all blood establishments in Xizang Zizhiqu had been officially operated, and 452 blood establishments nationwide had been put into operation. With the continuous improvement of the basic conditions, construction facilities, equipment and instruments of the blood establishments, as well as the increasing number and restructuring of blood services personnel, the proportion of highly educated health technicians was increased. In April 2018, the Blood Center of Xizang Zizhiqu initiated blood nucleic acid testing. So far, 31 provinces, autonomous regions, municipalities and Xinjiang Production and Construction Corps had maintained the ability of nucleic acid testing, and the ability of guaranteeing blood safety in China had stepped into a new stage.

IV. Blood Quality Management System was Improved Continuously, and the Quality Management Level of Blood Testing was Promoted

China had established a blood quality management system covering the whole process of blood collection and supply, and formed a relatively complete EQA system of blood collection and supply institutions, as well as clinical blood transfusion compatibility testing. The EQA system of blood collection and supply institutions basically covered the routine testing work of blood collection and supply institutions, and the results of various evaluation projects in 2018 remained stable. The EQA system of clinical blood transfusion compatibility testing had covered 31 provinces, autonomous regions and municipalities in China. In 2018, 5 EQA projects of the national evaluation-participation units all passed the quality evaluation test, playing an important role in ensuring blood safety.

V. Law Enforcement and Supervision of Blood Safety was Implemented at All Levels, and Prevention and Control Measures of Blood Safety were Continuously Optimized

In order to raise the awareness of blood safety, implement the responsibility of blood safety, and ensure the supply and safety of blood for clinical use, the National Health Commission randomly selected some blood collection and supply institutions and hospitals in 10 provinces (autonomous regions and municipalities directly under the central government) to carry out the technical verification of blood safety. At the same time, the Health Administrative Departments and the Health Supervision and Law Enforcement Departments of all provinces (autonomous regions and municipalities directly under the central government) regularly and irregularly supervised and inspected the blood collection and supply institutions and hospitals in accordance with the relevant provisions of the state. A top-down, comprehensive and unified law enforcement and supervision system was formed, ensuring that the blood collection and supply system operated coordinating to the laws and regulations, improving the evaluation system of blood collection and supply institutions, timely rectifying the found potential safety hazards, which further guaranteed the safety of blood donors and users.

VI. Capacity of Clinical Blood Use Management was Improved Continuously, and New Technologies and Methods were Promoted

The Health Administrative Departments of the country and provinces (autonomous regions and municipalities directly under the central government) continuously strengthened the management of clinical blood use from the channels of system, such as industry standard, new organization access, etc. Under the guidance of Health Administrative Departments at all levels, the system construction of clinical blood transfusion quality control centers at all levels was continuously improved. The quality control centers of clinical blood transfusion at all levels focused on the quality management means, such as evaluation, supervision, management and assessment of clinical rational use of blood, as well as the promotion of new technologies, personnel training and other work. On the one hand, the clinical safe use of blood was strengthened. On the other hand, under the condition of continuous increase of in-patient volume and operation volume, the related indexes of clinical blood consumption, such as blood consumption of per operation, blood consumption of per discharge, proportion of blood transfusion patients, blood consumption of per blood transfusion patient, platelet consumption of per operation and so on, all showed a downward trend, and the clinical blood consumption became more reasonable.

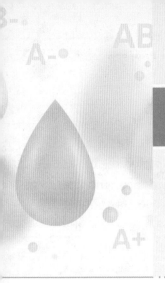

Chapter Two

Challenges

I. Blood Supply Still Faced Challenges

In recent years, with the continuous promotion of the Strategy of Healthy China , the average life expectancy had continued to increase, which further brought about the aging of the population; the number of elderly lying-in women increased with the full implementation of the Two-child policy, the medical service volume continued to rise with the improvement of the medical security level etc, which had put forward new and higher level of blood supply requirements. At present, China's blood supply was still in a state of "tight balance". There was still a gap between developed countries in terms of blood donation rate per thousand people and other indicators, and the contradiction between blood supply and demand still faces challenges.

II. The Independent Capacity of Blood Collection and Supply in Remote Areas Needed to be Improved

With the great attention and support of governments at all levels, blood collection and supply in the border areas continued to develop. However, due to the late start of blood collection and supply in the border areas, the social atmosphere of voluntary non-remunerated blood donation still needed to be fostered, and the security mechanism to be enhanced. At the same time, affected by the traditional concepts, the enthusiasm of the minority citizens to donate blood voluntarily was not high, and the majority of the voluntary non-remunerated blood donors were Han people. In addition, the blood collection and supply institutions in border areas had been faced with the problems of insufficient health technical talents, low overall quality of the talent team and brain drain. The talent problem was still one of the key factors restricting the development of blood collection and supply capacity in the border areas. Therefore, there were still challenges in improving the ability of blood supply and guarantee in the border areas.

III. Blood Safety Risks Still Existed

In 2018, dengue fever, a pathogen transmitted by blood transfusion, broke out in some areas of southern China, which indicated that China still faced a challenge in the prevention and control of new and recurrent blood-borne pathogens. At present, there was still a gap in the screening of blood-borne pathogens between China and countries like in Europe or Japan. The detection of infectious disease markers related to local and time-limited transfusion was still lack of larger samples from multiple centers and epidemiological data. In terms of blood screening technology, most of the in vitro diagnostic reagents used for blood screening in China are imported reagents, and there was still a certain gap between domestic reagents and imported reagents in terms of sensitivity, specificity and product stability.

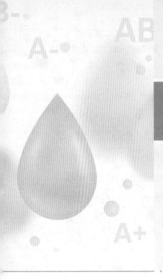

Chapter Three

Future Prospects

I. The Long-term Mechanism of Voluntary Non-remunerated Blood Donation was Explored

Voluntary non-remunerated blood donation is a medical and health cause with profound social significance. Local governments at all levels needed to further improve the long-term effective working mechanism of "government leadership, department cooperation, and the participation of the whole society" in voluntary non-remunerated blood donation to effectively shoulder the important responsibility of ensuring and improving people's livelihood. Financial investment was increased and the infrastructure of blood establishments was improved, which ensured that blood establishment's service systems were compatible with the development of health care. A salary system, which was compatible with the development of blood establishment's staff, was built. The training and development of professional and technical talents was strengthened. At the same time, the mechanism was innovated, the incentive measures of publicity and recruitment of voluntary non-remunerated blood donation were explored, and a social atmosphere to promote the value of voluntary non-remunerated blood donation was formed, which constantly expanded the team of blood donors.

II. The Blood Collection and Supply System Optimized

At present, most of the blood establishments in China were small, but comprehensive in function, making it difficult to retain talents and lower the operation cost. Referring to the experience of developed countries and the suggestion of the World Health Organization, actively exploring "decentralized collection, unified preparation and centralized detection" was an effective way to solve this problem. Through well-operated fixed blood collection sites and newly-set mobile blood collection sites, the service and capacity was enhanced continuously, and the blood supply was further guaranteed. It further strengthened laboratory facilities, ensured staffing, reduced operating costs and improved the blood quality by conducting blood component preparation in a unified way on a regional basis and launching blood concentrated test in on a provincial basis.

III. Refined Management of Blood Collection and Supply was Improved

It was expected to establish the overall quality management of blood collection and supply institutions, accelerate the building of national network of blood management information and improve the blood management information construction covering the whole process of blood collection and supply and clinical use, so as to strengthen the standardization and refined management of blood. It was also required to explore the "high quality, efficient and convenient" blood station service mode, reasonably plan the regional layout of blood establishment business, optimize business process, and improve service satisfaction. It was suggested to strengthen the service consciousness, standardize the service behavior, improve the service quality, raise the sense of acquirement of blood donors, and further ensure the quality and safety of blood.

IV. Standardized Management of Clinical Rational Blood Use

The work of Patient Blood Management (PBM) was further promoted, and the standardized management of clinical rational blood use was improved. The evaluation of clinical blood use was carried out, further improving the scientific and reasonable use of blood. The system of supervision, management and notification for the clinical use of blood was enhanced, and new technologies for rational use of blood were promoted, which was to reduce unnecessary blood transfusion, achieve the targeted clinical use of blood, maximize the quality and efficiency, and save blood resources.

V. Early Warning Mechanism for Blood Safety Risks was Established.

The monitoring of adverse reactions in blood transfusion was gradually augmented, and to build an early warning mechanism for blood safety was built in China, which was to prevent and block the possible blood safety risks in advance. A unified blood transfusion safety monitoring system and blood safety early warning mechanism was built, and the reporting system of transfusion adverse reactions in blood transfusion was improved, which was expected to strengthen the ability and level of diagnosis, categorization, classification, treatment and prevention of transfusion adverse reactions, reduce the occurrence of transfusion adverse reactions, and improve the safety of patients.

Appendices

Appendix 1   Summary of blood donation rate per 1,000 population in 2018

No.	Area	/per 1,000 population	Year on Year	
			/per 1,000 population	Growth Rate /%
1	Beijing	16.3	−1.0	−5.8
2	Tianjin	12.2	0.6	5.5
3	Hebei	10.6	0.4	4.1
4	Shanxi	9.9	0.6	6.7
5	Nei Mongol	8.7	0.4	4.3
6	Liaoning	9.8	−0.2	−2.1
7	Jilin	9.9	0.4	3.7
8	Heilongjiang	9.9	0.3	2.6
9	Shanghai	14.8	0.0	−0.1
10	Jiangsu	13.0	0.6	4.4
11	Zhejiang	12.5	0.4	3.4
12	Anhui	7.8	0.1	0.8
13	Fujian	8.7	0.0	−0.1
14	Jiangxi	8.6	0.5	6.3
15	Shandong	10.3	0.2	2.0
16	Henan	12.3	0.6	5.2
17	Hubei	11.6	0.3	2.9
18	Hunan	8.6	0.1	1.0
19	Guangdong	12.0	−0.1	−1.0
20	Guangxi	11.2	0.2	1.5

Continued

No.	Area	/per 1,000 population	Year on Year	
			/per 1,000 population	Growth Rate /%
21	Hainan	11.3	0.2	2.0
22	Chongqing	11.1	0.1	0.5
23	Sichuan	9.3	0.3	3.5
24	Guizhou	10.2	0.4	4.4
25	Yunnan	10.1	0.7	7.3
26	Xizang	0.5	−0.5	−49.9
27	Shaanxi	12.3	0.3	2.7
28	Gansu	8.1	0.0	−0.4
29	Qinghai	7.6	−0.2	−2.4
30	Ningxia	9.4	−0.4	−4.0
31	Xinjiang	6.3	−0.2	−2.7
32	Corps	5.8	−0.6	−10.0

Appendix 2   Summary of the volume of blood donation in 2018

No.	Area	Whole Blood			Platelet		
		/K U	Year on Year		/K TU*	Year on Year	
			/K U	Growth Rate/%		/ K TU*	Growth Rate/%
1	Beijing	506	−36	−6.6	88	−16	−15.5
2	Tianjin	289	14	5.0	55	4	8.8
3	Hebei	1,365	49	3.7	108	7	7.4
4	Shanxi	654	35	5.6	40	11	36.8
5	Nei Mongol	364	14	3.9	21	2	10.0
6	Liaoning	706	−16	−2.3	53	−1	−1.0
7	Jilin	424	17	4.1	28	2	8.5
8	Heilongjiang	637	17	2.8	37	1	3.6
9	Shanghai	457	−8	−1.6	45	4	8.5
10	Jiangsu	1,528	76	5.2	164	14	9.4

Continued

No.	Area	Whole Blood			Platelet		
		/K U	Year on Year		/K TU*	Year on Year	
			/K U	Growth Rate/%		/ K TU*	Growth Rate/%
11	Zhejiang	1,003	48	5.0	97	10	12.0
12	Anhui	764	3	0.3	37	4	12.8
13	Fujian	529	5	1.0	37	2	5.4
14	Jiangxi	637	35	5.8	43	6	15.9
15	Shandong	1,667	10	0.6	128	6	5.4
16	Henan	2,107	100	5.0	159	17	12.1
17	Hubei	1,037	27	2.6	103	14	16.0
18	Hunan	979	1	0.1	68	16	30.5
19	Guangdong	1,980	13	0.7	158	5	3.5
20	Guangxi	890	22	2.5	47	2	5.1
21	Hainan	162	7	4.2	11	1	8.7
22	Chongqing	519	2	0.4	29	2	7.6
23	Sichuan	1,240	37	3.1	50	7	17.0
24	Guizhou	563	34	6.4	27	6	27.1
25	Yunnan	725	74	11.4	36	9	31.6
26	Xizang	2	−2	−48.1	0	0	—
27	Shaanxi	766	10	1.4	43	9	27.5
28	Gansu	308	1	0.3	14	2	16.5
29	Qinghai	81	0	0.3	27	24	812.9
30	Ningxia	116	−3	−2.9	5	−1	−18.5
31	Xinjiang	245	−1	−0.3	21	3	19.4
32	Corps	28	−2	−7.1	1	0	−12.6

*TU: Treatment Unit

Appendix 3   Summary of individual blood donation rate in 2018

No.	Area	/%	Year on Year	
			/pct.	Growth Rate/%
1	Beijing	70.3	8.1	13.0
2	Tianjin	85.1	−1.7	−1.9
3	Hebei	78.5	−1.7	−2.1
4	Shanxi	80.3	−1.1	−1.3
5	Nei Mongol	85.2	3.4	4.2
6	Liaoning	77.1	−0.7	−0.9
7	Jilin	70.6	−0.7	−0.9
8	Heilongjiang	83.1	0.3	0.4
9	Shanghai	35.5	−1.5	−4.1
10	Jiangsu	64.1	1.3	2.1
11	Zhejiang	51.8	3.4	7.0
12	Anhui	78.7	−1.0	−1.2
13	Fujian	60.5	3.3	5.7
14	Jiangxi	65.9	−1.8	−2.6
15	Shandong	80.6	−2.7	−3.2
16	Henan	83.1	−3.0	−3.5
17	Hubei	87.6	−0.9	−1.0
18	Hunan	71.7	4.4	6.5
19	Guangdong	59.1	6.1	11.6
20	Guangxi	74.6	2.5	3.5
21	Hainan	63.5	2.8	4.6
22	Chongqing	84.4	6.1	7.8
23	Sichuan	62.8	−1.7	−2.7
24	Guizhou	83.5	7.1	9.3
25	Yunnan	64.7	−1.1	−1.7
26	Xizang	44.4	19.0	74.7
27	Shaanxi	84.4	−3.8	−4.4
28	Gansu	70.6	−4.4	−5.9
29	Qinghai	83.9	1.7	2.0
30	Ningxia	83.8	−13.7	−14.1
31	Xinjiang	84.4	−0.4	−0.4
32	Corps	99.2	4.8	5.0

pct.: percentage point

Appendix 4　Summary of 400ml blood donation rate in 2018

No.	Area	/%	Year on Year	
			/pct.	Growth Rate/%
1	Beijing	67.8	−5.0	−6.9
2	Tianjin	79.0	−1.8	−2.3
3	Hebei	81.0	−1.7	−2.1
4	Shanxi	90.0	−0.4	−0.4
5	Nei Mongol	67.1	−0.9	−1.3
6	Liaoning	74.9	−0.4	−0.5
7	Jilin	55.5	2.1	3.9
8	Heilongjiang	80.9	0.3	0.4
9	Shanghai	36.8	−1.2	−3.3
10	Jiangsu	38.6	2.0	5.5
11	Zhejiang	37.9	0.9	2.4
12	Anhui	50.7	−1.8	−3.4
13	Fujian	49.0	1.7	3.7
14	Jiangxi	57.8	0.1	0.2
15	Shandong	63.0	−3.9	−5.8
16	Henan	92.6	−0.5	−0.6
17	Hubei	49.8	0.5	0.9
18	Hunan	54.0	−0.1	−0.2
19	Guangdong	45.1	0.4	0.9
20	Guangxi	59.4	−0.2	−0.3
21	Hainan	52.3	1.4	2.8
22	Chongqing	54.5	−1.4	−2.4
23	Sichuan	50.5	−1.6	−3.1
24	Guizhou	56.3	1.7	3.1
25	Yunnan	34.7	9.0	34.9
26	Xizang	5.2	1.0	24.0
27	Shaanxi	67.3	−2.4	−3.4
28	Gansu	33.3	0.4	1.3
29	Qinghai	81.0	3.7	4.7
30	Ningxia	83.0	−2.3	−2.7
31	Xinjiang	54.9	0.2	0.4
32	Corps	37.7	−2.2	−5.6

Appendix 5　Summary of female blood donor rate in 2018

No.	Area	/%	Year on Year	
			/pct.	Growth Rate/%
1	Beijing	30.7	2.4	8.4
2	Tianjin	25.6	0.6	2.5
3	Hebei	33.4	0.8	2.3
4	Shanxi	30.2	−0.1	−0.2
5	Nei Mongol	34.7	−0.5	−1.3
6	Liaoning	39.6	0.4	1.0
7	Jilin	36.7	0.7	1.8
8	Heilongjiang	40.5	−0.3	−0.7
9	Shanghai	30.4	0.3	1.2
10	Jiangsu	39.4	0.6	1.5
11	Zhejiang	38.3	0.5	1.2
12	Anhui	40.4	0.3	0.7
13	Fujian	37.8	0.9	2.5
14	Jiangxi	39.0	0.7	1.7
15	Shandong	29.6	0.8	2.9
16	Henan	37.0	−0.2	−0.4
17	Hubei	38.1	0.8	2.1
18	Hunan	39.6	1.8	4.9
19	Guangdong	31.6	0.9	2.8
20	Guangxi	34.9	1.0	2.9
21	Hainan	30.8	1.0	3.2
22	Chongqing	50.6	0.8	1.6
23	Sichuan	48.1	1.2	2.5
24	Guizhou	51.4	2.0	4.1
25	Yunnan	44.7	2.4	5.8
26	Xizang	25.7	0.2	0.9
27	Shaanxi	37.7	1.2	3.3
28	Gansu	31.1	1.0	3.2
29	Qinghai	33.8	0.8	2.3
30	Ningxia	36.5	0.5	1.4
31	Xinjiang	33.9	1.5	4.7
32	Corps	34.7	1.9	5.7

Appendix 6　Summary of blood donation rate aged 18 to 35 in 2018

No.	Area	/%	Year on Year	
			/pct.	Growth Rate/%
1	Beijing	64.9	−2.0	−3.1
2	Tianjin	70.5	0.1	0.2
3	Hebei	46.1	−1.1	−2.3
4	Shanxi	42.9	−0.8	−1.7
5	Nei Mongol	45.8	−1.0	−2.1
6	Liaoning	48.0	−0.2	−0.3
7	Jilin	50.3	0.3	0.6
8	Heilongjiang	40.9	−0.7	−1.7
9	Shanghai	73.3	0.0	0.0
10	Jiangsu	50.9	−1.1	−2.2
11	Zhejiang	53.7	−0.6	−1.2
12	Anhui	52.0	−0.2	−0.5
13	Fujian	52.2	−1.1	−2.0
14	Jiangxi	56.1	0.5	0.9
15	Shandong	52.6	0.1	0.3
16	Henan	40.1	−0.2	−0.6
17	Hubei	52.9	−0.4	−0.7
18	Hunan	54.5	0.0	0.1
19	Guangdong	63.6	0.2	0.4
20	Guangxi	53.7	0.2	0.4
21	Hainan	63.0	−0.2	−0.3
22	Chongqing	49.6	−1.2	−2.4
23	Sichuan	43.0	−1.6	−3.6
24	Guizhou	56.2	0.1	0.2
25	Yunnan	60.6	1.7	2.9
26	Xizang	68.8	−5.3	−7.1
27	Shaanxi	54.0	0.2	0.3
28	Gansu	58.1	−0.8	−1.4
29	Qinghai	46.0	1.0	2.2
30	Ningxia	55.3	−1.3	−2.3
31	Xinjiang	57.4	2.3	4.2
32	Corps	57.0	0.2	0.4

Appendix 7　Summary of blood donation rate with bachelor degree or above in 2018

No.	Area	/%	Year on Year	
			/pct.	Growth Rate/%
1	Beijing	34.6	7.9	29.4
2	Tianjin	23.0	2.8	13.7
3	Hebei	15.3	1.1	7.4
4	Shanxi	19.1	−0.5	−2.5
5	Nei Mongol	23.2	1.6	7.6
6	Liaoning	21.0	0.3	1.6
7	Jilin	24.2	1.6	7.2
8	Heilongjiang	21.3	−0.3	−1.2
9	Shanghai	23.4	2.2	10.3
10	Jiangsu	21.5	0.3	1.3
11	Zhejiang	22.2	−0.3	−1.5
12	Anhui	24.6	1.1	4.8
13	Fujian	29.1	1.1	3.8
14	Jiangxi	25.5	1.3	5.4
15	Shandong	19.8	1.2	6.6
16	Henan	13.7	1.5	12.1
17	Hubei	27.1	1.1	4.3
18	Hunan	28.8	0.6	2.2
19	Guangdong	19.3	1.2	6.4
20	Guangxi	18.3	−0.2	−0.9
21	Hainan	28.8	0.7	2.3
22	Chongqing	21.0	0.7	3.7
23	Sichuan	17.2	0.2	0.9
24	Guizhou	15.9	−1.6	−9.2
25	Yunnan	24.3	2.5	11.5
26	Xizang	21.4	−2.3	−9.7
27	Shaanxi	21.7	1.4	6.7
28	Gansu	19.5	0.7	3.5
29	Qinghai	19.6	1.0	5.5
30	Ningxia	20.0	2.4	13.6
31	Xinjiang	19.8	0.5	2.4
32	Corps	26.4	2.4	10.2

Appendix 8　Summary of blood testing at blood centers in 2018

No.	Area	Testing number			Ineligible number			Ineligible rate	
		/TPT*	Year on Year		/TPT*	Year on Year		/%	Year on Year/pct.
			/TPT*	Growth Rate/%		/TPT*	Growth Rate/%		
1	Beijing	412	-30	-6.9	61	-5	-7.3	14.8	-0.1
2	Tianjin	218	10	4.9	28	-1	-4.0	12.6	-1.2
3	Hebei	898	35	4.0	104	0	0.3	11.5	-0.4
4	Shanxi	420	20	5.0	62	-4	-6.2	14.7	-1.8
5	Nei Mongol	223	4	1.7	24	-3	-12.3	10.8	-1.7
6	Liaoning	587	85	17.0	80	-3	-3.9	13.6	-2.9
7	Jilin	298	7	2.4	31	-2	-5.9	10.6	-0.9
8	Heilongjiang	414	10	2.4	44	0	0.4	10.5	-0.2
9	Shanghai	279	-4	-1.4	41	-2	-5.5	14.8	-0.7
10	Jiangsu	1,117	49	4.6	95	3	3.1	8.5	-0.1
11	Zhejiang	811	-4	-0.5	107	2	1.9	13.1	0.3
12	Anhui	526	24	4.7	43	-2	-4.8	8.1	-0.8
13	Fujian	386	1	0.3	56	-3	-4.3	14.6	-0.7
14	Jiangxi	429	23	5.7	38	-4	-9.8	8.9	-1.5
15	Shandong	1,110	37	3.4	97	4	3.9	8.7	0.0
16	Henan	1,277	57	4.7	126	2	1.4	9.9	-0.3

Continued

No.	Area	Testing number			Ineligible number			Ineligible rate	
		/TPT*	Year on Year		/TPT*	Year on Year		/%	Year on Year/pct.
			/TPT*	Growth Rate/%		/TPT*	Growth Rate/%		
17	Hubei	699	38	5.8	41	4	10.2	5.9	0.2
18	Hunan	619	13	2.1	43	-2	-4.8	6.9	-0.5
19	Guangdong	1,472	52	3.7	182	12	6.8	12.4	0.4
20	Guangxi	611	36	6.2	62	0	0.2	10.2	-0.6
21	Hainan	121	5	4.3	19	2	13.5	15.4	1.2
22	Chongqing	388	8	2.2	56	-2	-3.0	14.4	-0.8
23	Sichuan	852	24	2.9	105	1	0.6	12.3	-0.3
24	Guizhou	395	27	7.3	38	4	11.4	9.7	0.4
25	Yunnan	548	51	10.4	71	15	26.5	12.9	1.6
26	Xizang	3	-2	-42.6	1	-1	-27.3	50.1	10.5
27	Shaanxi	510	12	2.4	43	-6	-11.5	8.5	-1.3
28	Gansu	225	-2	-0.7	23	-6	-20.4	10.1	-2.5
29	Qinghai	57	2	4.4	12	3	28.4	21.6	4.0
30	Ningxia	73	1	1.8	11	0	2.0	15.5	0.0
31	Xinjiang	176	-1	-0.5	22	0	-0.2	12.6	0.0
32	Corps	20	-1	-4.2	3	0	-16.1	12.8	-1.8

*TPT: Thousand Person-Time

Appendix 9　Summary of pre-donation blood screening in 2018

No.	Area	Screening number			Ineligible number			Ineligible rate	
		/TPT*	Year on Year		/TPT*	Year on Year		/%	Year on Year/pct.
			/TPT*	Growth Rate/%		/TPT*	Growth Rate/%		
1	Beijing	412	-30	-6.9	54	-4	-6.5	13.1	0.0
2	Tianjin	218	10	4.9	25	-1	-2.3	11.6	-0.9
3	Hebei	898	35	4.0	93	3	2.9	10.4	-0.1
4	Shanxi	420	20	5.0	53	-4	-6.8	12.7	-1.6
5	Nei Mongol	223	4	1.7	19	-3	-13.2	8.5	-1.5
6	Liaoning	587	85	17.0	73	-2	-2.9	12.5	-2.6
7	Jilin	298	7	2.4	27	-2	-5.3	9.2	-0.8
8	Heilongjiang	414	10	2.4	38	1	1.8	9.1	0.0
9	Shanghai	279	-4	-1.4	28	0	0.0	10.0	0.1
10	Jiangsu	1,117	49	4.6	81	4	5.8	7.3	0.1
11	Zhejiang	811	-4	-0.5	97	3	2.8	11.9	0.4
12	Anhui	526	24	4.7	32	0	0.3	6.2	-0.3
13	Fujian	386	1	0.3	49	-1	-1.6	12.6	-0.2
14	Jiangxi	429	23	5.7	30	-4	-11.2	7.1	-1.4
15	Shandong	1,110	37	3.4	79	5	6.4	7.1	0.2
16	Henan	1,277	57	4.7	108	1	1.3	8.4	-0.3

Continued

No.	Area	Screening number			Ineligible number			Ineligible rate	
		/TPT*	Year on Year		/TPT*	Year on Year		/%	Year on Year/pct.
			/TPT*	Growth Rate/%		/TPT*	Growth Rate/%		
17	Hubei	699	38	5.8	27	5	25.3	3.9	0.6
18	Hunan	619	13	2.1	29	0	-1.0	4.7	-0.1
19	Guangdong	1,472	52	3.7	140	14	10.9	9.5	0.6
20	Guangxi	611	36	6.2	49	2	4.2	8.1	-0.2
21	Hainan	121	5	4.3	16	2	14.6	13.0	1.2
22	Chongqing	388	8	2.2	47	1	1.7	12.0	-0.1
23	Sichuan	852	24	2.9	77	4	5.2	9.0	0.2
24	Guizhou	395	27	7.3	27	6	28.8	6.9	1.2
25	Yunnan	548	51	10.4	59	16	36.6	10.8	2.1
26	Xizang Zizhiqu	3	-2	-42.6	1	0	-25.8	47.8	10.8
27	Shaanxi	510	12	2.4	35	-4	-11.0	6.8	-1.0
28	Gansu	225	-2	-0.7	19	-5	-22.0	8.3	-2.3
29	Qinghai	57	2	4.4	11	3	36.1	19.6	4.6
30	Ningxia	73	1	1.8	11	0	4.6	14.5	0.4
31	Xinjiang	176	-1	-0.5	18	0	1.1	10.5	0.2
32	Corps	20	-1	-4.2	2	0	-18.2	9.9	-1.7

*TPT: Thousand Person-Time

Appendix 10　Summary of blood laboratory testing at blood centers in 2018

No.	Area	Testing number			Ineligible number			Ineligible rate		
		/K	Year on Year		/K	Year on Year		/%	Year on Year	
			/K	Growth Rate/%		/K	Growth Rate/%		/%	Year on Year/pct.
1	Beijing	365	-20	-5.1	7	-1	-13.1	1.9	-0.2	
2	Tianjin	189	10	5.3	2	-1	-19.3	1.2	-0.4	
3	Hebei	800	36	4.6	10	-2	-18.1	1.3	-0.4	
4	Shanxi	377	25	7.0	9	0	-2.4	2.3	-0.2	
5	Nei Mongol	229	10	4.7	5	-1	-9.0	2.2	-0.3	
6	Liaoning	427	-12	-2.6	6	-1	-13.9	1.5	-0.2	
7	Jilin	269	8	3.2	4	0	-9.7	1.5	-0.2	
8	Heilongjiang	379	12	3.3	6	0	-7.6	1.5	-0.2	
9	Shanghai	348	-3	-0.7	13	-2	-15.5	3.8	-0.7	
10	Jiangsu	1,047	48	4.8	13	-2	-11.0	1.3	-0.2	
11	Zhejiang	710	47	7.1	10	-1	-6.1	1.4	-0.2	
12	Anhui	497	8	1.7	10	-2	-17.7	2.1	-0.5	
13	Fujian	343	2	0.7	8	-2	-18.1	2.3	-0.5	
14	Jiangxi	395	23	6.2	8	0	-4.0	1.9	-0.2	
15	Shandong	1,039	12	1.2	18	-1	-5.9	1.7	-0.1	
16	Henan	1,211	65	5.7	19	0	1.8	1.6	-0.1	

Continued

No.	Area	Testing number			Ineligible number			Ineligible rate	
		/K	Year on Year		/K	Year on Year		/%	Year on Year/pct.
			/K	Growth Rate/%		/K	Growth Rate/%		
17	Hubei	719	22	3.2	14	-2	-10.2	2.0	-0.3
18	Hunan	596	12	2.0	14	-2	-12.0	2.3	-0.4
19	Guangdong	1,410	62	4.6	42	-2	-5.2	2.9	-0.3
20	Guangxi	601	0	0.0	13	-2	-12.6	2.2	-0.3
21	Hainan	105	3	3.1	3	0	7.6	2.8	0.1
22	Chongqing	342	6	1.8	9	-3	-21.5	2.7	-0.8
23	Sichuan	768	28	3.8	29	-3	-10.1	3.7	-0.6
24	Guizhou	398	16	4.1	11	-2	-16.4	2.8	-0.7
25	Yunnan	486	37	8.3	11	-1	-8.8	2.3	-0.4
26	Xizang	1	-2	-54.6	0	0	-48.5	4.5	0.5
27	Shaanxi	475	17	3.6	9	-1	-13.4	1.8	-0.4
28	Gansu	213	-2	-0.8	4	-1	-11.9	1.9	-0.2
29	Qinghai	48	0	-0.5	1	0	-17.5	2.4	-0.5
30	Ningxia	65	-2	-3.3	1	0	-27.4	1.0	-0.3
31	Xinjiang	179	-19	-9.4	4	0	-6.2	2.1	0.1
32	Corps	1.8	0	-2.0	1	0	-7.8	3.3	-0.2

Appendix 11   Summary of blood component separation rate in 2018

No.	Area	/%	Year on Year	
			/pct.	Growth Rate/%
1	Beijing	100.00	0.00	0.00
2	Tianjin	99.82	0.01	0.01
3	Hebei	99.69	0.10	0.10
4	Shanxi	99.71	0.07	0.07
5	Nei Mongol	99.32	−0.01	−0.01
6	Liaoning	99.87	0.03	0.03
7	Jilin	99.87	0.06	0.06
8	Heilongjiang	99.02	−0.31	−0.31
9	Shanghai	99.86	0.07	0.07
10	Jiangsu	99.97	0.02	0.02
11	Zhejiang	99.88	0.02	0.02
12	Anhui	99.86	0.08	0.08
13	Fujian	99.97	0.02	0.02
14	Jiangxi	100.00	0.01	0.01
15	Shandong	99.90	0.02	0.02
16	Henan	99.82	−0.08	−0.08
17	Hubei	99.94	0.01	0.01
18	Hunan	100.00	0.01	0.01
19	Guangdong	99.98	0.02	0.02
20	Guangxi	99.99	0.00	0.00
21	Hainan	100.00	0.00	0.00
22	Chongqing	99.67	−0.23	−0.23
23	Sichuan	99.98	0.07	0.07
24	Guizhou	99.94	−0.03	−0.03
25	Yunnan	100.00	0.00	0.00
26	Xizang	97.86	10.45	11.95
27	Shaanxi	99.92	0.02	0.02
28	Gansu	99.77	0.03	0.03
29	Qinghai	99.60	−0.07	−0.07
30	Ningxia	97.22	−2.73	−2.73
31	Xinjiang	96.80	−3.16	−3.16
32	Corps	97.69	−2.11	−2.11

Appendix 12   Summary of concentrated platelet separation rate in 2018

No.	Area	/%	Year on Year	
			/pct.	Growth Rate/%
1	Beijing	6.2	3.8	153.1
2	Tianjin	10.6	3.6	50.4
3	Hebei	0.2	0.2	64,224.7
4	Shanxi	0.8	0.0	4.0
5	Nei Mongol	8.4	3.3	64.6
6	Liaoning	0.0	−0.1	−100.0
7	Jilin	0.9	−1.9	−68.7
8	Heilongjiang	0.2	0.1	161.1
9	Shanghai	0.9	−0.1	−5.3
10	Jiangsu	0.2	0.1	36.1
11	Zhejiang	0.2	0.2	1,121.8
12	Anhui	5.0	0.4	8.7
13	Fujian	1.0	1.0	—
14	Jiangxi	0.6	0.2	46.2
15	Shandong	0.0	0.0	—
16	Henan	0.2	0.0	−7.0
17	Hubei	0.1	0.1	—
18	Hunan	9.1	1.0	11.9
19	Guangdong	7.7	3.8	97.2
20	Guangxi	2.6	0.1	4.8
21	Hainan	0.0	0.0	—
22	Chongqing	0.0	0.0	28.5
23	Sichuan	7.1	0.4	5.9
24	Guizhou	1.0	−0.8	−44.4
25	Yunnan	0.0	0.0	−75.3
26	Xizang	0.0	0.0	—
27	Shaanxi	1.3	−0.4	−22.9
28	Gansu	0.0	0.0	−6.2
29	Qinghai	6.4	1.5	29.2
30	Ningxia	0.8	−2.4	−75.8
31	Xinjiang	0.5	0.1	36.5
32	Corps	0.1	−0.5	−87.9

Appendix 13　Summary of total blood supply volume in 2018

No.	Area	/K U	Year on Year	
			/K U	Growth Rate/%
1	Beijing	1,281	23	1.8
2	Tianjin	662	44	7.2
3	Hebei	2,511	77	3.2
4	Shanxi	1,062	72	7.3
5	Nei Mongol	657	69	11.8
6	Liaoning	1,272	−35	−2.7
7	Jilin	788	24	3.2
8	Heilongjiang	1,227	122	11.0
9	Shanghai	900	13	1.5
10	Jiangsu	3,125	209	7.2
11	Zhejiang	2,231	131	6.2
12	Anhui	1,421	3	0.2
13	Fujian	971	4	0.4
14	Jiangxi	1,249	70	6.0
15	Shandong	3,118	10	0.3
16	Henan	4,073	191	4.9
17	Hubei	1,947	67	3.6
18	Hunan	2,071	4	0.2
19	Guangdong	4,459	903	25.4
20	Guangxi	1,650	8	0.5
21	Hainan	279	9	3.3
22	Chongqing	998	92	10.2
23	Sichuan	2,086	−19	−0.9
24	Guizhou	1,022	97	10.5
25	Yunnan	1,357	180	15.3
26	Xizang	10	2	33.1
27	Shaanxi	1,462	19	1.3
28	Gansu	1,376	801	139.3
29	Qinghai	186	0	0.0
30	Ningxia	224	−10	−4.3
31	Xinjiang	518	60	13.2
32	Corps	84	26	45.7

Appendix 14　Summary of platelet use volume (10,000 people) in 2018

No.	Area	/K TU*	Year on Year	
			/K TU*	Growth Rate/%
1	Beijing	522.1	32.5	6.6
2	Tianjin	371.4	34.9	10.4
3	Hebei	142.7	10.3	7.8
4	Shanxi	89.5	11.8	15.2
5	Nei Mongol	105.8	26.1	32.7
6	Liaoning	120.2	−2.5	−2.0
7	Jilin	102.2	5.8	6.0
8	Heilongjiang	97.2	5.0	5.4
9	Shanghai	196.5	10.3	5.5
10	Jiangsu	195.7	16.6	9.3
11	Zhejiang	172.4	18.1	11.7
12	Anhui	64.8	7.1	12.2
13	Fujian	95.2	6.7	7.5
14	Jiangxi	91.1	10.2	12.6
15	Shandong	127.3	7	5.8
16	Henan	166.1	17.8	12.0
17	Hubei	171.3	23.2	15.6
18	Hunan	109.8	24.3	28.4
19	Guangdong	151.7	12.4	8.9
20	Guangxi	99.7	5.6	5.9
21	Hainan	120.1	10.3	9.3
22	Chongqing	90.6	7.6	9.1
23	Sichuan	69.5	9.7	16.3
24	Guizhou	78.7	15.8	25.2
25	Yunnan	74.3	18.5	33.3
26	Xizang	00.0	0.0	—
27	Shaanxi	113.4	24	26.9
28	Gansu	50.8	9.3	22.5
29	Qinghai	446.4	−37.2	−7.7
30	Ningxia	77.6	−15.1	−16.2
31	Xinjiang	73.0	2.0	2.7
32	Corps	29.8	−3.5	−10.5

*TU: Treatment Unit

Appendix 15　Summary of tangible components utilization rate in 2018

No.	Area	/%	Year on Year /pct.	Growth Rate/%
1	Beijing	106.2	3.8	3.7
2	Tianjin	110.4	3.6	7.8
3	Hebei	99.8	0.2	0.5
4	Shanxi	100.5	0.1	0.2
5	Nei Mongol	107.7	3.3	5.4
6	Liaoning	99.9	0.0	−0.1
7	Jilin	100.7	−1.9	−3.5
8	Heilongjiang	99.2	−0.2	−0.3
9	Shanghai	100.8	0.0	0.0
10	Jiangsu	100.2	0.1	0.1
11	Zhejiang	100.1	0.2	0.5
12	Anhui	104.9	0.5	0.9
13	Fujian	101.0	1.0	1.9
14	Jiangxi	100.6	0.2	0.4
15	Shandong	99.9	0.0	0.1
16	Henan	100.0	−0.1	−0.2
17	Hubei	100.0	0.1	0.1
18	Hunan	109.1	1.0	2.0
19	Guangdong	107.6	3.8	7.0
20	Guangxi	102.6	0.1	0.2
21	Hainan	100.0	0.0	0.0
22	Chongqing	99.7	−0.2	−0.4
23	Sichuan	107.1	0.5	0.8
24	Guizhou	100.9	−0.8	−1.4
25	Yunnan	100.0	0.0	−0.1
26	Xizang	97.9	10.4	15.6
27	Shaanxi	101.2	−0.4	−0.7
28	Gansu	99.8	0.0	0.1
29	Qinghai	106.0	1.4	3.1
30	Ningxia	98.0	−5.1	−9.8
31	Xinjiang	97.3	−3.0	−5.8
32	Corps	97.8	−2.6	−5.2

Appendix 16　Summary of physical discarded blood in 2018

No.	Area	Physical discarding			Discarding rate	
		/K U	Year on Year		/%	Year on Year
			/K U	Growth Rate/%		/pct.
1	Beijing	3.3	0.3	10.2	0.3	0.0
2	Tianjin	2.7	0.7	38.4	0.4	0.1
3	Hebei	90.1	10.2	12.8	3.4	0.3
4	Shanxi	106.3	16.1	17.9	8.9	0.7
5	Nei Mongol	54.0	-1.5	-2.7	7.5	-1.0
6	Liaoning	76.2	-3.0	-3.8	5.6	-0.1
7	Jilin	5.8	1.5	33.5	0.7	0.2
8	Heilongjiang	5.2	-0.7	-11.8	0.4	-0.1
9	Shanghai	16.7	1.1	7.3	1.8	0.1
10	Jiangsu	4.0	-0.6	-12.5	0.1	0.0
11	Zhejiang	39.3	3.1	8.6	1.7	0.0
12	Anhui	113.1	17.2	17.9	7.2	1.0
13	Fujian	57.4	-8.2	-12.5	5.4	-0.7
14	Jiangxi	43.6	8.2	23.1	3.3	0.5
15	Shandong	5.7	-0.7	-11.1	0.2	0.0
16	Henan	58.9	1.4	2.4	1.4	0.0

Continued

No.	Area	Physical discarding			Discarding rate	
		/KU	Year on Year		/%	Year on Year
			/KU	Growth Rate/%		/pct.
17	Hubei	88.9	7.8	9.6	4.3	0.2
18	Hunan	50.7	-10.0	-16.5	2.3	-0.5
19	Guangdong	233.9	-51.7	-18.1	4.9	-2.3
20	Guangxi	69.9	12.1	21.0	4.0	0.7
21	Hainan	0.2	0.0	17.7	0.1	0.0
22	Chongqing	22.6	2.4	12.0	2.2	0.0
23	Sichuan	171.8	-14.1	-7.6	7.3	-0.5
24	Guizhou	49.5	-15.1	-23.4	4.5	-1.8
25	Yunnan	77.5	7.3	10.4	5.3	-0.2
26	Xizang	0.2	0.0	3.3	2.0	-0.5
27	Shaanxi	6.6	-3.5	-34.5	0.4	-0.2
28	Gansu	20.5	-3.4	-14.4	1.5	-2.5
29	Qinghai	1.2	0.3	36.1	0.6	0.2
30	Ningxia	4.4	1.3	40.7	1.9	0.6
31	Xinjiang	29.8	3.0	11.3	5.3	-0.1
32	Corps	2.1	0.1	2.5	2.4	-0.9

Appendix 17   Summary of blood collection in major cities in 2018

City	Blood donation rate/per 1,000 population	Blood collection volume per donor/ml	Platelet collection volume per donor/Unit per 10,000 population
Beijing	16.4	5.5	40.9
Tianjin	12.2	4.4	35.4
Shijiazhuang	17.7	6.5	30.8
Taiyuan	24.1	9.1	36.5
Hohhot	10.1	3.4	18.5
Shenyang	14.1	5.2	24.9
Changchun	14.9	5.0	23.7
Harbin	14.4	5.3	21.0
Shanghai	14.8	4.1	18.6
Nanjing	22.7	7.3	51.6
Hangzhou	18.2	5.6	40.9
Hefei	14.7	4.5	17.7
Fuzhou	11.2	3.9	19.6
Nanchang	20.3	6.8	26.3
Jinan	18.4	6.1	32.1
Zhengzhou	23.4	8.4	63.3
Wuhan	20.3	6.6	64.3
Changsha	19.5	7.0	31.1
Guangzhou	25.3	8.1	46.7
Nanning	18.6	6.1	27.4
Haikou	27.1	8.7	45.2
Chongqing	11.0	3.5	8.7
Chengdu	13.9	4.8	23.1
Guiyang	21.0	6.5	29.0
Kunming	25.0	8.3	38.8
Lhasa	2.7	0.6	—
Xi'an	18.3	6.4	30.2
Lanzhou	16.1	4.9	27.7

Continued

City	Blood donation rate/per 1,000 population	Blood collection volume per donor/ml	Platelet collection volume per donor/Unit per 10,000 population
Xining	15.6	7.8	112.1
Yinchuan	18.4	6.9	20.9
Ürümqi	15.5	4.7	37.4
Shenzhen	12.9	4.5	22.2
Dalian	12.2	3.9	17.5
Qingdao	12.7	4.4	20.4
Ningbo	11.5	3.4	14.7
Xiamen	13.8	4.0	19.4